HORSES
THAT SAVE
LIVES

Also by the Author:

The Legendary Appaloosa

HORSES
THAT SAVE
LIVES

True Stories of Physical, Emotional, and Spiritual Rescue

CHERYL DUDLEY

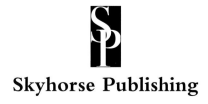

Skyhorse Publishing

Skyhorse Publishing books may be purchased in bulk at special discounts for sales promotion, corporate gifts, fund-raising, or educational purposes. Special editions can also be created to specifications. For details, contact the Special Sales Department, Skyhorse Publishing, 555 Eighth Avenue, Suite 903, New York, NY 10018 or info@skyhorsepublishing.com.

www.skyhorsepublishing.com

10 9 8 7 6 5 4 3 2 1

Library of Congress Cataloging-in-Publication Data

Dudley, Cheryl.
  Horses that save lives : true stories of physical, emotional, and spiritual rescue / Cheryl Dudley.
     p. cm.
   ISBN 978-1-60239-721-7 (alk. paper)
  1. Horses--Psychological aspects. 2. Horsemen and horsewomen--Psychology. 3. Horse owners--Biography. 4. Human-animal relationships. 5. Lifesaving. I. Title.
   SF301.D83 2009
   636.1--dc22
                                    2009018686

Printed in China

CONTENTS

INTRODUCTION

If it were possible to capture the essence of the horse in one comprehensive sentence, what would it say? I'm not talking about the beauty or elegance of the animal, for many poets have captured his physical attributes in fine lines of poetry.

What I'm talking about is the abstract, unseen power that draws us to him, the hidden heart and soul of an animal that longs to connect with humankind, an animal that throughout the centuries has suffered at our hands, yet time and again has mercifully forgiven and saved us. Is it possible to sum up that essence in one short sentence?

Perhaps the best description on the power of the horse I've come across is in the poem "Equus Caballus," written by Joel Nelson. This poem gives credence to the horse, who gave us not only mobility and utility, but also the ability to conquer nations and thrive as civilizations. It captures the heroism of this humble yet powerful animal and his willingness to look past our abuses, mistakes, and shortcomings and love us unconditionally.

Here are the words to that powerful poem:

Equus Caballus

I have run on middle fingernail through Eolithic morning.

I have thundered down the coach road with the Revolution's warning.

I have carried countless errant knights who never found the grail.

I have strained before the caissons, I have moved the nation's mail.

I've made knights of lowly tribesmen and kings from ranks of peons.

I have given pride and arrogance to riding men for eons.

I have grazed among the lodges and the tepees and the yurts.

I have felt the sting of driving whips, lashes, spurs and quirts.

I am roguish—I am flighty—I am inbred—I am lowly.

I'm a nightmare—I am wild—I am the horse.

I am gallant and exalted—I am stately—I am noble.

I'm impressive—I am grand—I am the horse.

I have suffered gross indignities from users and from winners,

I have felt the hand of kindness from the losers and the sinners.

I have given for the cruel hand and given for the kind.

Heaved a sigh at Appomattox when surrender had been signed.

I can be as tough as hardened steel—as fragile as a flower.

I know not my endurance and I know not my own power.

I have died with heart exploded 'neath the cheering in the stands—

Calmly stood beneath the hanging noose of vigilante bands.

I have traveled under conqueror and underneath the beaten.

I have never chosen sides—I am the horse.

The world is but a players' stage—my roles have numbered many.

Under blue or under gray—I am the horse.

So I'll run on middle fingernail until the curtain closes,

And I will win your Triple Crowns and I will wear your roses.

Toward you who took my freedom I've no malice or remorse.

I'll endure—This Is My Year—I am the Horse!

Joel, who lives in Alpine, Texas, is one of today's most respected poets and reciters. His CD, *The Breaker in the Pen*, is the only cowboy poetry recording ever nominated for a Grammy Award.

Without a doubt, the horse continues to capture our attention and play a significant role in contemporary life. Those who have the honor of experiencing the power of the horse are often changed forever.

Every horse-human relationship is unique. Down through the centuries, millions of humans would attribute their very reason for living to their best horse friend. As Joel Nelson's poem attests, the horse has given more to humankind than we can begin to comprehend. His gift to us includes companionship and sometimes even life itself.

The consensus among many horse lovers is that horses give them hope and a reason to get up in the morning. The more I talk to horse lovers, particularly those who have encountered difficult times in life, the more I hear this one line, this one commonality among them, that makes them so strongly bonded to their horse:

"My horse saved my life."

Amazingly, the salvation for these horse lovers was often physical—and it sometimes happened more than once. But oftentimes the salvation came in a more abstract form.

"My horse saved me from suicide."

"My horse gave me hope to go on when nothing else could."

"My horse helped me recover from cancer; helped me recover emotionally from a divorce; helped me get me feet back on the ground."

"My horse gave me a reason to keep on going."

This book is about that one-line sentence that captures the essence of a regal, beautiful, and powerful animal that has the ability to reach deep into our souls and save us. This is about the horses that saved lives.

Many of the stories are of a physical nature—when danger or death was imminent—and it is only because a horse interceded that these storytellers are alive. Other stories capture that other plane of salvation—the emotional salvation that drove our storytellers back to sanity and a clear mind and keeps them functioning on a solid plane. The voices in this book range from a Vietnam veteran and persons with disabilities to show ring queens and everyday horse owners.

The horse has no favorites. He never takes sides. He just gives and gives unconditionally. Now step with me into the world of humble horses—those heroes who no more know their power than their ability to protect, heal, and give hope to the lost.

HORSES
THAT SAVE
LIVES

BOLD THE DREAM HORSE

— *Melissa Godin* —

The German philosopher Goethe wrote,
"Whatever you can do, or dream you can, begin it!
Boldness has genius, power, and magic in it."

When I was a child I loved horses, but my mother never allowed me to ride because she was afraid I would get hurt. So instead I read horse books and eventually acquired quite a collection: *Black Beauty*, *The Black Stallion*, *Misty of Chincoteague*, and others.

My father was an avid fan of horseracing, and through him I became familiar with the greats. He remembered seeing Man of War run, as well as War Admiral, Whirlaway, Citation, and many others. Sometimes we would go out to the local racetrack, bring out the folding chairs, and watch the horses thunder around the clubhouse turn. He took great pride in my ability as an eight-year-old to recite the list of all the Kentucky Derby winners since its beginning in 1875.

That is the one wonderful memory I have of my father. But my childhood was very difficult because my parents fought often and hard; they eventually divorced when I was fifteen. My father passed on shortly thereafter. I couldn't bring friends to the house because of the fighting, so books became my closest friends. When I was about eighteen years old, I had a job and did ride horses a few times; I also fell off a few times. I didn't ride again for many, many years. I married and had a family, but I never lost my love for horses. Whether I was driving by a field, attending a horse show, or going to the county fair, I always looked at them longingly.

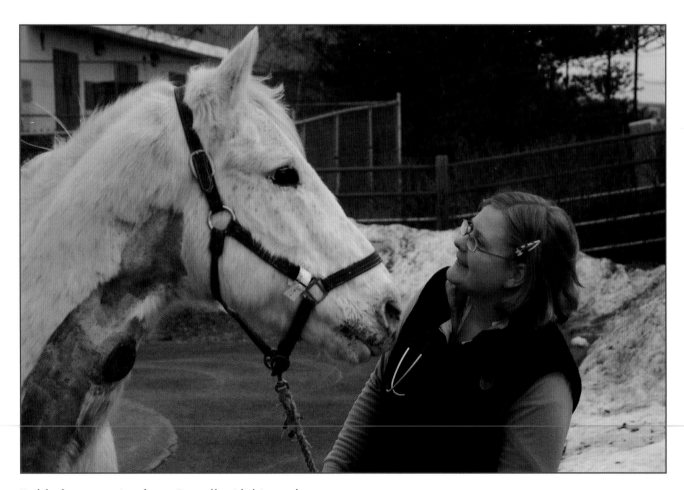

Bold after returning from Cornell with his tracheotomy

In December 2000 I was diagnosed with a malignant melanoma in the lymph nodes. There was no primary site on the skin, and it was only discovered when one of the nodes swelled up to the size of a golf ball. The prognosis was dire: sixteen percent chance of survival with surgery and a year of chemotherapy. At the time I had two teenage daughters and had just gone back to school to get my bachelor's degree in special education.

The year of chemo was brutal. There were times I felt great strength and promise and many times when I was in the depths of despair. At the six-month point, I remember telling my husband, Rick, that I just couldn't go on any longer. I wanted to give up. I was in so much pain and at the end of my emotional rope.

But that was before I had the dream.

I fell asleep one night in the midst of physical and emotional turmoil. Perhaps it was the chemo that prompted the dream—perhaps not. I like to believe it was more of a vision. It was extremely vivid, with all of the sights, sounds, and bodily sensations associated with the waking world. As I fell into slumber, I was immersed in a horrendous rolling, boiling, sickly yellow light, and it felt as if a green shroud was descending on me. I couldn't run. There was nowhere to go, and it felt as if I was cemented in place.

Suddenly out of this cloud a pure white horse materialized and came toward me and lay down in front of me. I walked toward the horse and lay down against his belly. All sensations of fear and pestilence evaporated, and I was filled with an overwhelming feeling of light, peace, and hope.

When I finally woke up, I felt like all was well. I knew I could go on. I can't say that I was given the assurance that I would live, but I knew I was given the gift of healing.

After the cancer treatments ended, it seemed like a blessing and a curse. I began to feel better and regain my strength. I saw the world like Dorothy in *The Wizard of Oz*, like I had been living in Kansas and now, with the world bright and beautiful around me, I was in living in Oz. It was the spring of 2002, and I felt new life emerging in me.

The white horse from my vision was never far from my thoughts.

As any cancer survivor will tell you, there is always a malignant fear of "what if." What if the cancer comes silently back? During that period of time, the book about Seabiscuit by Laura Hillenbrand came out. In the book a seemingly broken-down horse and a trainer, owner, and jockey—each carrying great sadness and disappointment—meet and bring Seabiscuit to the heights of racing glory in the 1930s, despite adversity and heartbreak. The first time I saw the movie in the theater, I was transfixed. I remember walking out of the theater, totally unable to speak because the emotion was so great. I went back to see the movie several times and felt the power of his story anew. The final lines in the movie inspired and strengthened me: The jockey says that everybody thinks they found a broken-down horse and fixed him, but in truth it was the horse that fixed them all.

So often we look to people for inspiration, hope, and strength. I found myself dwelling on all the stories my father had told me about the racing greats. They inspired me to finish my own race—whatever the odds. One thing that cancer teaches you is that we don't have forever. All of those times we tell someone we'll do something today or tomorrow are empty promises. We just don't know.

During my emotional healing, I decided to return to my childhood dream of riding horses. But there was one major obstacle: I was deathly afraid to get on a horse and reluctant to even stand near one. Perhaps my mother taught me well, or I had watched too many movies, but three years passed before I could make myself do it. By then I was fifty-five, which made this endeavor seem even more ridiculous or foolhardy. Nonetheless, I found a trainer, and the "fun" began.

My trainer always said that my biggest obstacle was my fear and that she had never seen anyone so fearful who at the same time wanted something so badly. I kept on with my lessons and never did really graduate to the canter. My trainer kept referring to it as the C-word. I would make faltering attempts but never got more than halfway around the ring. And then the day came when I fell off and couldn't ride for twelve weeks. But my love transcended my fear and I went back. One day, though, my trainer, exasperated with my attempts, said, "Perhaps you don't have the courage to ride." It broke my heart.

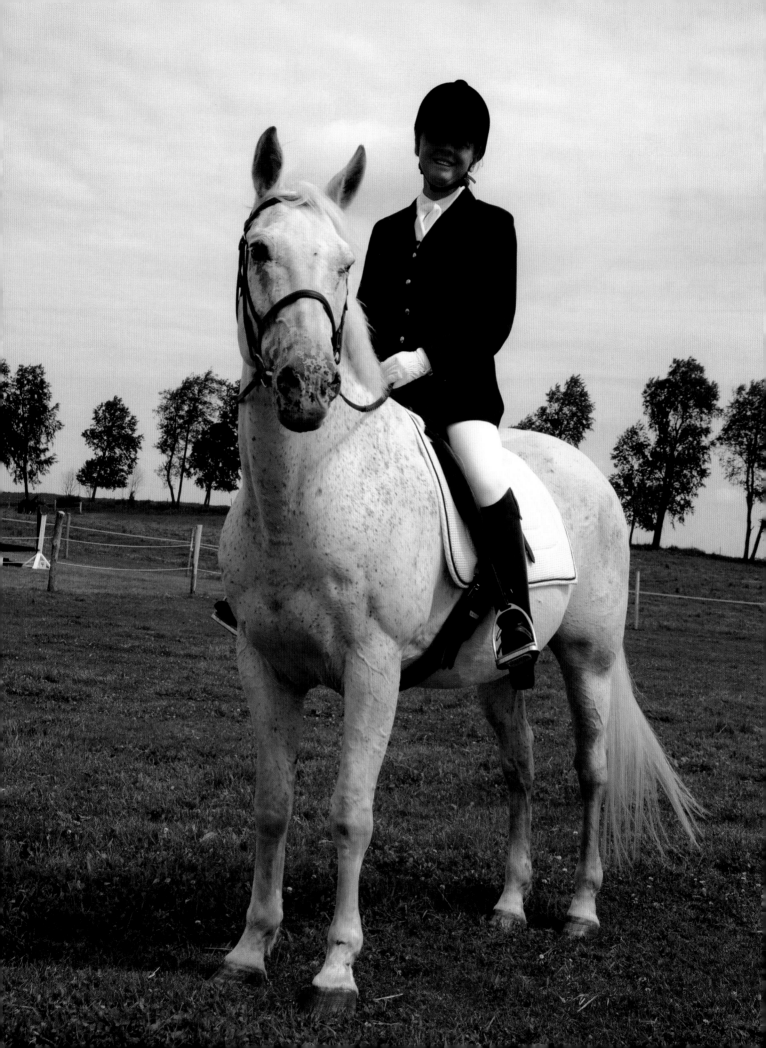

In 2008, I became friends with a woman who boarded her horse at a nearby stable. She convinced me to ride with her and I agreed, not knowing how it would utterly change my life.

At the new stable I was introduced to the horse in my dream. He was a twenty-four-year-old pure white Appaloosa named Bold. We made an instant connection. He stood tall in his winter coat as I mounted him and did a walk-trot around the ring.

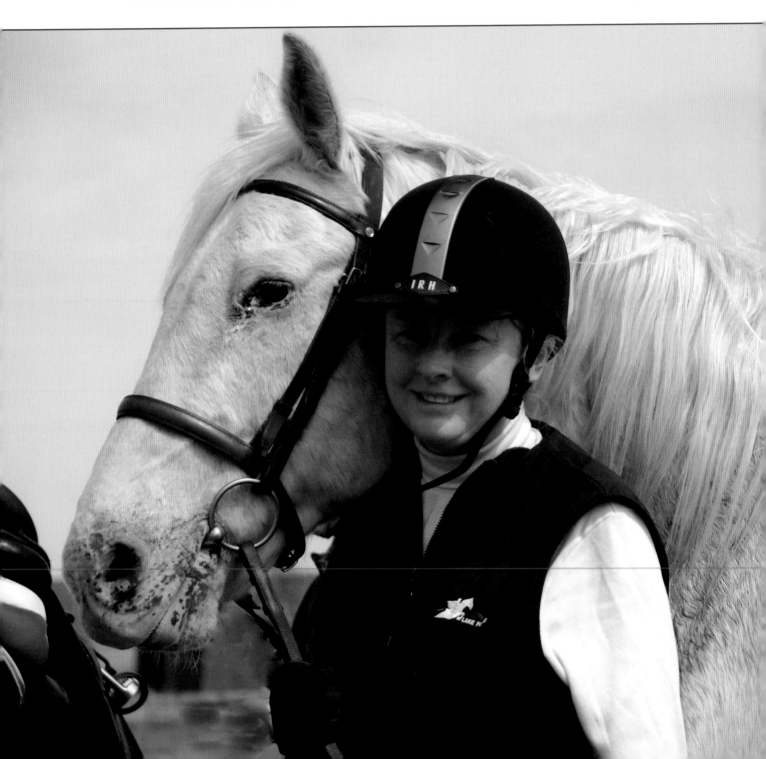

The trainer knew my story and my failed efforts to canter, so she didn't push me—she just suggested I try.

I don't remember thinking anything, but I immediately shortened the reins, pressed with my legs, and off we went around a very tiny enclosed area. There was no protest, no waiting, and no "I can't"—we just went.

The words don't exist to explain why this occurred. The best I can say is that the feeling I had in my dream of the white horse was there when I mounted Bold.

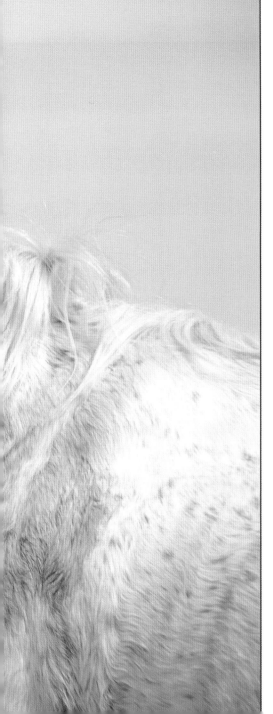

The German philosopher Goethe wrote, "Whatever you can do, or dream you can, begin it! Boldness has genius, power, and magic in it." In a matter of a few months, Bold and I had won five blue ribbons for dressage and walk-trot-canter classes. We even jumped rails. Bold would like to go three feet, but I'm only game for eighteen inches. Take him out of the show ring, and he's always up for a trail ride. The best thing about him is his disposition; nothing riles him. Coming out of the show ring one day a cat and a dog came screaming down the pathway. Bold simply kicked out his back legs and didn't bolt, but two horses a few feet away threw their riders. It seems ironic that the horse who has given me the gifts of courage, hope, and healing is named Bold.

In June 2008, Bold and I went into the show ring and won another blue ribbon. It was shortly after that the owners came to me and told me they were going to retire Bold. Momentarily I felt my world crash beneath my feet. That is, until they said, "We want you to have him." When the owners gave him to me, they said it was because it was a match made in heaven; little did they know that I believe I met him long before I ever rode him.

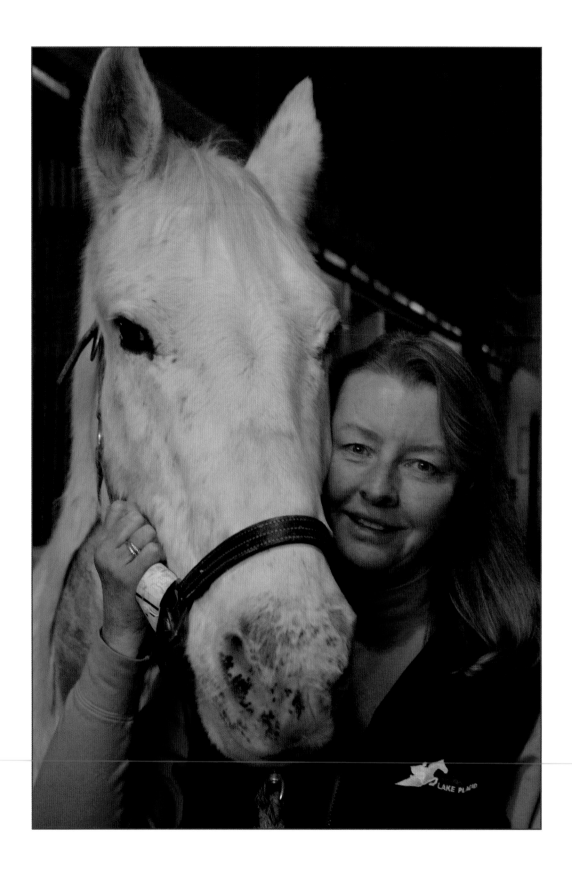

Cancer gave me new life, and my horse has been my teacher. I have learned to live in the present moment, something every rider knows is a necessary element in horsemanship. I had lived my life continually looking to the past with regret and to the future with fear. Now I know that I have the power inherent in every moment to determine the course of my future and to not be adrift on the waters of chance.

Bold has taught me that every dream is possible given love, persistence, and determination. Those years I spent looking longingly at riders and their horses and the many pictures and figurines I have of white horses are now my reality. I have learned that passion is the impetus, the mover of our dreams. I have learned that we only need to take the first step and then continue to put our feet in front of us, taking measured steps, no matter how large or small, toward our goal. We have to know, not think, that our dream can become a reality.

I remember when people asked me why I didn't have my own horse. I would answer that I did; he was out there, and when the time and circumstances were right we would be brought together. I liken it to a flower unfolding in its own time, as it is with a dream.

My horse has taught me to be joyful in all and through all. In the years since my illness, our family has gone through hardship and illness. At the present time we have two elderly parents under hospice care. I have learned that we may be surrounded by sadness or harmony, but if we can find the one thing that deeply fulfills us, that emanates from our soul, it will give light to our world. Joseph Campbell, noted scholar and mythologist, is famous for saying, "Follow your bliss. Find where it is, and don't be afraid to follow it." I found my bliss on my horse, in the barn, and out in the pasture.

Cancer can be seen as an enemy, a thief of all that we hold dear in life. I say that it can also be the bearer of great gifts. The poet Rumi wrote:

◄ Melissa and Bold

This being human is a guest house.

Every morning a new arrival.

A joy, a depression, a meanness,

Some momentary awareness comes as an unexpected visitor.

Welcome and entertain them all!

Even if they're a crowd of sorrows who violently sweep your house

empty of its furniture.

Still, treat each guest honorably.

He may be clearing you out

For some new delight.

I have been transformed. I have seen a dream made real. I have seen a sad past that no longer has any power over me. This is the new delight that came when cancer swept clean my house. I can say with certainty that I never would have attempted to ride had two white horses as teachers not come into my life. When my time on earth is complete, I will look back at Bold with love and gratitude for the way he saved my life.

Update

On December 7, 2008, Bold was out in the field while the farm managers were busy feeding the horses. All of a sudden he started to run wildly, flailing his head in obvious distress. All hands rushed to the field and saw that he had blood spurting out of his nose. They saw very quickly that Bold was not able to breathe, and it looked as though he had minutes to live. Upstate New York is rural and large-animal vets are few. There wasn't time to contact any and have them arrive quickly.

But at that exact moment, the local vet came down the driveway on a social call. She immediately jumped into action. She found two washing machine tubes and put them into Bold's nose and down into his lungs. His condition stabilized but was critical. Melissa arrived shortly after and found a pathetic horse: tired, muddy, and bloody. It seemed very likely that the only alternative was euthanasia.

Melissa asked the vet if Bold had a chance. She said yes. "I'm going to give him that chance then," Melissa replied.

Cornell Equine Hospital was a three-and-a-half hour drive, and it was imperative that Bold be taken there as quickly as possible. Miracle number two comes into play. The vet had been working on her green card, and the paperwork had been going on for months. Two days before Bold's emergency, she received word that everything was finalized, and she was able to practice veterinary medicine in the United States. This enabled her to call Cornell and put plans in place for his arrival. Although it was questionable as to whether or not Bold would survive that long drive, he was loaded into the van, and they began what would be a six-hour journey through a nor'easter.

"We drove through treacherous road conditions with whiteouts, cars off the road, traffic stopped on the other side, but, like the parting of the Red Sea, six hours later we arrived at Cornell," said Melissa.

At Cornell, doctors performed a tracheotomy and found that Bold's larynx was paralyzed. Doctors have not discovered the cause, despite every test in the book. Bold responded well to the tracheotomy. Before long he was eating, drinking, and flirting with a stablemate.

During this time, Melissa had another dream. Bold had the operation and she was in an unknown town walking the streets. Suddenly she somehow got word that Bold was racing that day.

"I rushed back and saw him in a river with other horses just as if he were racing on the track," said Melissa. "Bold was struggling to keep his head above water. I remember hearing myself shouting, "No, no, no" and then I woke up.

Bold's former owner, who had him from a yearling, had recently contacted Melissa and told her that one of the sires in his pedigree was Bold Ruler, the sire of Secretariat.

After eight weeks at Cornell, Bold the Wonder Horse came home. Melissa continues to believe in dreams.

ABU KHAN

— Donna Borba —

"Abu started getting scared. He knew something was not right. I tried to stay calm, but I was terrified."

When Donna Borba of Escalon, California, was a little girl, she used to pester her parents continuously to take her on those little pony rides at the fair. She knows her parents hoped the infatuation would wear off eventually, but it never did. Not only did she love riding ponies, she just couldn't stop thinking about horses in general. She owned a favorite Breyer horse named Thunderbolt that she was in love with, and that fulfilled her dreams—sort of—until she was ten years old.

In 1970, Donna's dreams came true. Her uncle Kenneth, who was involved in the Arabian Horse Association, gave her a full-blooded Arabian horse named Abu Khan.

Her uncle prepared Abu for showing, but the horse seemed to be somewhat of an oddity in the Arabian world, with a stocky conformation more like a Quarter Horse.

"Abu was a misfit, just like me," said Donna.

Donna's parents didn't own a place to keep horses at the time, but Donna saw Abu Khan every summer until she was fourteen years old and he was four. Until then, her uncle took him to shows and trained him for her. Then, when she was fourteen, her parents bought a place with acreage to keep horses, and Donna was finally able to take her horse home.

"Abu Khan was my world," said Donna. "I ate, drank, and did my homework with him. He could be cantankerous at times, but that was part of what made me love him so much."

Through the years, Donna and Abu formed an amazing friendship. When she was eighteen, Donna went to work for a Quarter Horse cutting ranch, where she trained cutting horses. She took Abu along and used him as a turn-back horse in the cutting pen. One day during a show, the judges pulled Donna aside and asked her what kind of horse Abu was, thinking he was at least part Quarter Horse because of his build.

"He's all Arabian," Donna said. The judges just stared at her in amazement. From that time on, Donna knew she owned a talented horse. She started team penning and winning with him, forging a bond that became stronger every year. That bond proved so valuable that Donna still finds some of the things Abu did for her hard to believe—times when extraordinary events occurred and the dedication of Abu became powerfully evident.

The first time Abu saved Donna's life, the two were trail riding with a group of friends down a steep, soft slope. For some unknown reason, some of the horses behind her spooked and started to run down the slope. Donna and Abu were out front—the worst possible location.

"My horse started to go down the slope too fast. So I got scared and just jumped off him," Donna said. "But what happened next still stuns me. The horses coming down the hill behind us started to fall. One knocked me down, and I couldn't get up. I just lay there waiting to get crushed or trampled." Time stood still. As

Donna closed her eyes and waited for the inevitable, she suddenly noticed a shadow over her.

"Abu was still close to me when I got off and was knocked down on the slope. I yelled when I went down—or screamed. The next thing I knew he was standing over the top of me and I was looking up at his belly, and the horses were slamming into him as they passed. It happened so fast. Then Abu stepped over me carefully, put his nose gently down to me, and then started off after the others. I screamed 'No! Abu!' I still remember the panic in my voice. That's when he put on the brakes, spun around, and came running back to me. By then I was on my feet. He came up to me and put his head in my chest. I still have a hard time believing it happened. I realized then how deeply devoted Abu was to my well-being."

The second time Abu saved Donna's life was a few years later. "I used to ride my horse from Hidden Valley, where my sister lived, to Agoura Hills, which is about fourteen miles," she said. "One day I was in a hurry and decided to take a shortcut. That decision could have taken my life if it hadn't been for Abu."

Donna really didn't know the mountain terrain well, but her instincts told her to go up a steep mountain and down the other side, which seemed like a fairly direct route home. "When I got to the top of the hill—there was no other side. It was practically a cliff. By now it was getting dark, and I didn't have time to turn back. Abu started to step down the other side, but he stumbled. I knew I couldn't stay on his back and make it down safely, so I tied the reins to the saddle and grabbed hold of Abu's tail. He safely walked us both down the hill, sliding all the way."

By the time Donna was twenty-one, she had learned to trust Abu completely. And the third time he saved her life, she really understood his amazing ability to read her mind. Again she was riding around in Agoura Hills when a car came up behind her and Abu and started following closely.

"Abu got real edgy, but there was no way out of the canyon because it was steep on both sides. The car was filled with strange men, and Abu started getting scared. He knew something was not right. I tried to stay calm, but I was terrified. I put my hand on Abu's neck to calm him while I searched frantically for a way out. We were all alone in the hills—there was no one else around for miles."

Suddenly Donna saw a narrow deer trail up ahead that led up the mountain. The problem was that the trail was across the road from where she and Abu were walking. This meant that they would have to somehow get far enough ahead of the car to cross in front of it.

"Abu saw the trail, too," said Donna. "As we neared it, his anxiety grew. He knew exactly what the plan was. I got this eerie feeling that he could read my mind."

By this time the men in the car were jeering at Donna, and she began to feel the real danger of her predicament. As Abu became more tense and edgy, Donna worked hard to keep him calm. "As soon as we got close enough to the trail, I took my hand off Abu's neck and he immediately sped up," said Donna. So did the car.

"We veered in front of the car dangerously close and hit the deer trail at full speed. Abu didn't stop running until we got to the top."

When the two reached the hilltop, Abu stopped, spun around, and let out a loud snort. The car below had stopped and the men were looking up at this magnificent Arabian horse. Abu, in his glory, with his head up and nostrils flared, gave out another loud snort at the awestruck men as if to say, "So there!"

"He was in his glory, and again I was in wonder at this amazing animal," said Donna.

"My Abu Khan lived to be thirty years old. He died in January 2000—and I still don't know how to deal with it," Donna said in tears. "He became the high point year-end world team penning champion in 1986. That was the year I quit showing. I thought it was best to end when we were both at the top. I just couldn't go into the arena without him.

"Horses are so honest. If I made mistakes, Abu always forgave me. When I was eighteen years old, I started training colts, and I've trained horses now for thirty years and have owned and trained many great horses. But Abu will always hold a special place in my heart. He taught me so much about patience and humility. I always counted on him. I was truly blessed to have known Abu Kahn."

THE MUSTANG PROJECT

— Murray Chico —

"I tried just about every drug I could find," said Murray.

But then he rediscovered horses.

You might say that Murray Chico has been given a second chance at life. At seventeen years old, he's already lived an extraordinarily challenging life marred by heartache, physical pain, and misfortune. But now he's serious about getting his life on track, specially equipped with the horses of the Mustang Project, operated by a man named Lee Kyser of Assurance Home in Roswell, New Mexico.

Murray was born on the Mescalero Apache Indian Reservation in New Mexico, the only child of his mother and father. When he was still a baby, his father was killed, and his mother eventually abandoned him to be raised by other family members. His mother had several other children over the years—half siblings to Murray. He has never gotten to know any of them.

You may think that living with family would be safe and nurturing, but for Murray it was dangerous and destructive. When he was seven years old and a student in teacher Cynthia Eggleston's second-grade class, she noticed some obvious problems with the young boy. After evidence of severe abuse surfaced, with her help he was removed from his aunt's home on the Mescalero Apache Reservation. The Egglestons went through the appropriate training to become foster parents and took Murray in as their own son.

"They were the only loving family I ever lived with," said Murray, who over the years has lived in three different foster homes. But even though he was in a

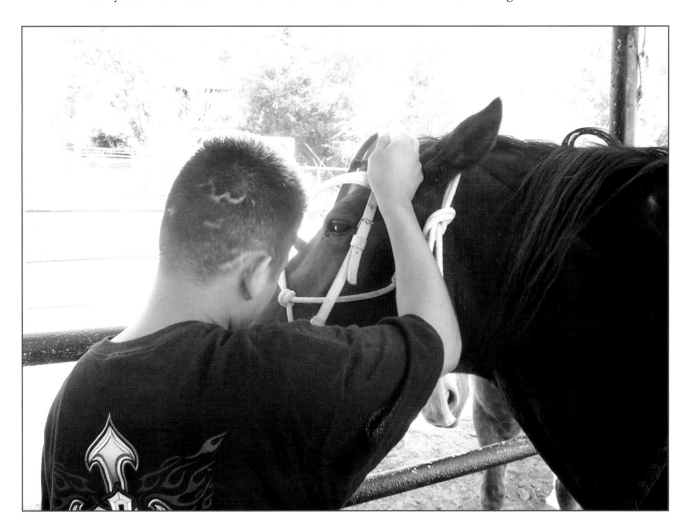

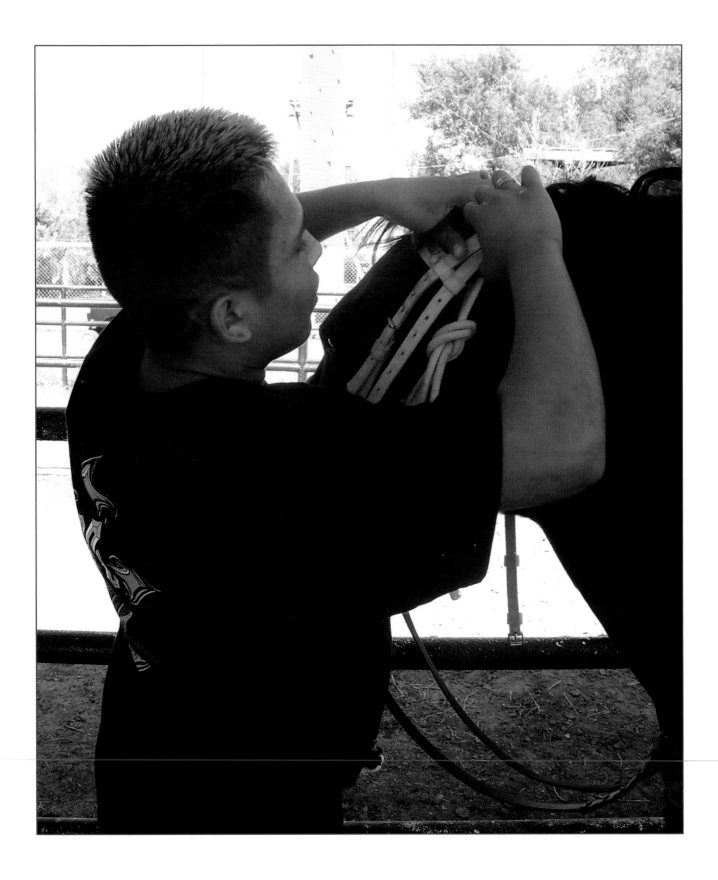

good home, Murray was plagued with anger and emotional problems because of the abuse he had suffered in his young life. He went through years of counseling and treatment centers. In some of the treatment centers he visited, he was introduced to hippotherapy, a form of treatment using horses. It was during these times that he was reminded of the one loving constant in his life: horses.

"My mother's family on the reservation had horses, and we did some rodeo when I was very little," said Murray. "Horses have always been there for me, when no one else was. Even back then I had this special connection with them."

After an episode of hospitalization when Murray was nine years old, childcare authorities decided that the boy should be placed in a different foster home. In spite of the fact that the Egglestons had been loving foster parents for nearly three years, authorities believed Murray would be best served living with a Native American family instead.

He went to his new home on March 17, 2001, marking another important turning point in the young boy's life. On March 18, the day after Murray arrived at his new home, he was left in the backyard with his new family's eleven-year-old German Shepherd–mix dog. Murray had been around dogs and wasn't afraid of them at all, so he decided to brush the dog out. As he gently stroked the dog with the brush, for some reason, the dog suddenly turned and attacked him. While the dog tore at Murray's face and neck, he screamed as best he could. His foster mother heard him and bolted to the backyard. She was almost too late. She found ten-year-old Murray bleeding profusely, with life-threatening injuries to his head, ear, and throat. The dog was taken away, and Murray was left to fight for his life.

Murray was rushed to the hospital and ended up in the pediatric intensive care unit with a grim prognosis: With the deep wounds to his throat, he may never be able to speak above a whisper. On top of that, he was denied visitation from the family that had cared for him for three years—the Egglestons, who frantically longed to see the boy they loved.

Murray was hospitalized for three months. The road to recovery was long and hard. He had to learn to walk, talk, and eat all over again.

Murray was released back into the Eggleston's custody, but by then his spirit was as wounded as his body. While his physical wounds slowly healed, his emotional wounds festered. Although he continued to receive therapy, deep down he became more angry and disturbed.

When he was a young teen, Murray was falsely accused of a crime and sent to jail for two years. When he was released, he was passed from one treatment center after another. His salvation was his chance to occasionally connect with horses. As soon as the opportunity arose, Murray began to abuse drugs and alcohol to escape the pain and anger he felt.

"I tried just about every drug I could find," he said.

But then when Murray was sixteen years old, he was sent to Assurance Home in New Mexico, where he met Lee Kyser—the man Murray says is like a father to him. He became involved in a horse program that would eventually put him on the road to freedom.

Lee Kyser has a long history of passion for horses. He began riding when he was four years old. He became a teacher, guidance counselor, and principal, while at the same time riding the New Mexico trails and team roping. After he retired as a school administrator, he directed an after-school program for kids until 1997, when he started working at Assurance Home.

Kyser operates a program at Assurance Home called the Mustang Project, where at-risk teens gentle and work with recently captured, green-broke Mustangs. These tough little horses eventually become therapeutic riding horses for handicapped riding programs around the country.

The challenge was just what young Murray needed, even though he didn't know it at the time.

"I wasn't cooperative at first," he said. "I still had a bad attitude and continued to get into trouble and mess around." So Murray ended up back in jail for another six months. From there, he was sent to another treatment center. Finally, at his last treatment center, Murray was attacked by some other boys, who broke his eye socket.

But that's not all that was broken. Murray Chico was finally ready to change, to cooperate with his treatment, and make his life better. In August 2008, Murray went back to Assurance Home to start working with the Mustangs again. This time things were different.

"Horses have always been my outlet," he said. "I knew that I could always talk to them and they understood. They never judged me, but just listened. They help me cope."

Involvement in the Mustang Project has offered Murray enormous opportunities to face and overcome the challenges he's encountered in life. He's learning patience, trust, self-awareness, and accomplishment, while also learning that he is unique and special. While helping himself, he's also helping others, giving him a deep sense of purpose and value. There are not many activities for youth that provide such opportunity.

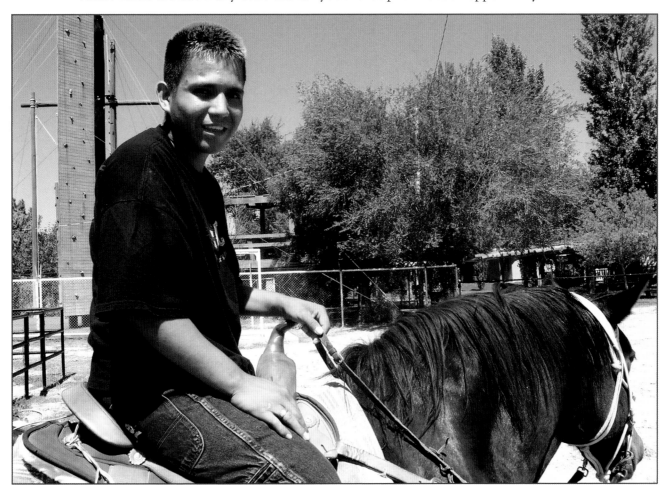

"Murray is an outstanding young man," said Ron Malone, director of Assurance Home. "All of us are crazy about him here. He's been through so much, yet he's such a great person."

Malone first heard of using troubled youth to gentle Mustangs at a hippotherapy conference he attended, where clinician Frank Bell gave a presentation. It was there that he became convinced the idea was perfect for Assurance Home. In 2000, Malone and Kyser picked up the first two Mustangs for their troubled youth.

Kyser claims that the horses help the children calm down and think about how to get what they want. They learn the value of patience and can all relate to the fact that the Mustangs were once wild and are now tame.

"Our youth understand how it feels to be mistreated," he said. "With the Mustang Project, they learn confidence, communication skills, and how to respond to the horse's needs."

Murray is working with a Mustang named Jeff right now. "I can't say that any particular horse has meant the most," he said. "All the horses that have come into my life through the years have given me hope and kept me going."

But one particular horse, perhaps, can exemplify Murray's life. It's a horse named Rosie, who was trained and went out for use but had to come back for further training. "That was a good experience for the kids because it taught them that it's always easier to start with a clean slate than with scars," said Kyser. "Murray has had some really bad experiences. Working with the horses helps him understand why he may have trouble building relationships with others."

Murray is considering a career in horsemanship and is even thinking about hippotherapy. "I want to spend my life working with the horses and helping people," he said. "I think that is a good ambition."

About the Mustang Project

The Mustang Project has been featured on CNN, CBS, *Western Horseman* magazine, and the *Albuquerque Journal*: www.assurancehome.org

HORSE ADDICTION: MY DRUG OF CHOICE

—— *Sue McMurray* ——

"Gypsy was there in the pasture with her thick mane I could brush and her little solid body that I could lean against when my dad was hurting and didn't want me around him in the house."

Two weeks before my fifth birthday in 1969, my family was involved in a serious car accident that left my sister a paraplegic and my father a quadriplegic. My mother was driving a new Opal Cadet when she hit black ice on Interstate 90 in Moses Lake, Washington, and lost control of the car. My mom and dad were driving my sister and her roommate back to Washington State University after Thanksgiving break. My family was unaware that mixing radial tires affected the steering capacity of the car, thus hindering the ability to successfully maneuver out of skid.

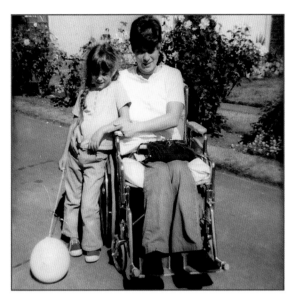

Sue at age five with her sister Kathy

I was playing at home with my ten-year-old brother, John, when the phone rang. My sister, Debra, who was fifteen, answered the phone and then came downstairs to where we were. She was crying. She said something like, "Mom, Dad, and Kath have been in an accident. Kath and Dad are hurt really bad!" John and I looked at each other for a moment, not comprehending the gravity of her emotional state. Then John said, "Oh, she's just lying! Let's go play!" And we ran off to resume our game.

This small, innocent moment of denial foreshadowed the way our family dealt with the ensuing crisis. It was like we took this enormous hit but we acted like nothing happened. In the following days, months, and years, we didn't talk about what any of us were feeling or that our lives were now changed forever.

I remember often being in a fearful and anxious state of mind. I had trouble sleeping. I had one recurring dream that our house was filling up with water, and I couldn't manage to push Kathy's and Dad's wheelchairs outside to safety. In another, a Sasquatch was stalking me in woods where I often played around our house. This was during the 1970s, when a few television newscasts reported some "sightings" of bigfoot near Packwood and the Mount Rainier area, not too far from where we lived. In the dream, I would run in agonizingly slow motion, trying to make it to the house to keep the predator from getting inside, where my family was sitting ducks.

When I started school, I was often nauseated, and I had a hard time handling my emotions. My report cards often had penned notes from my teachers that read "Needs improvement in self-control," which meant I often got upset and panicky in class over little things like forgetting to put my name on my paper before I handed it in. I was too afraid to ask for it back and risk seeing my teacher's disapproval.

Following the accident, I changed from happy and secure to withdrawn, depressed, and silent. Everyone in the family did what they could to help my mom deal with this terrible situation. I did my part by staying out of the way and becoming somewhat invisible. To this day, I am not comfortable being in the spotlight because of this childhood conditioning. As if there were not enough going on, my dad developed colon cancer that went undetected until it was already at stage four. He passed away five years after the accident, when I was ten.

Being around animals helped me cope with the extreme stress of this situation. I had several dogs that were a great source of comfort to me, but I always longed for a pony. My dream came true one night when my oldest brother, Dan, came home with a Shetland pony named Gypsy. Dan and I were always really close. As a young adult of twenty, he didn't have a lot of money, but he knew I loved horses and made special arrangements to get me that Shetland pony. It is one of the best memories I have.

Though Gypsy officially started my riding activities, she wasn't much for riding. A witherless wonder, Gypsy would run and put her head down so that I would slide right down her neck and fall off. She could bow her neck and charge straight through any one-rein stop I could attempt, but I didn't care. She was the inspiration for many drawings that replaced the words I didn't have to express my emotions and the sadness I felt most of the time. She was there in the pasture with her thick mane I could brush and her little solid body that I could lean against when my dad was hurting and didn't want me around him in the house.

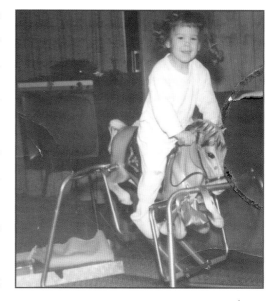

Gypsy was the stepping-stone to my next horse, Joe, a Quarter Horse gelding lent to me by a kind neighbor when I was ten, shortly after the funeral. I used Joe in 4-H, which helped me become a little more social and feel less different from my peers.

Joe served as a bridge to other, more challenging horses owned by Judi Hook, a hunter jumper coach

Sue at age three

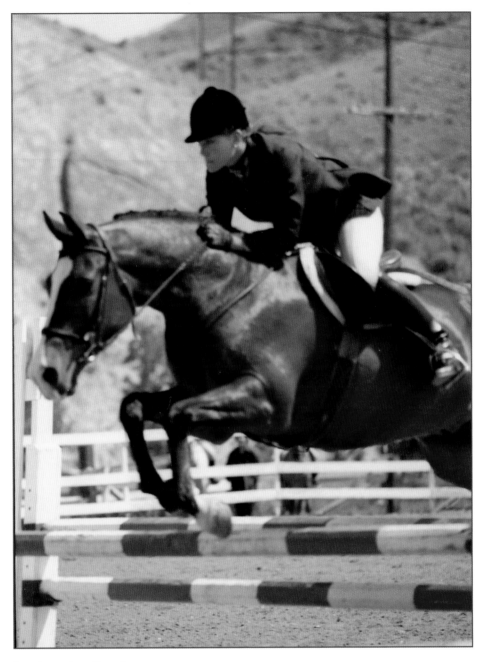

Sue jumping Reggie

who taught me, mostly for free, more advanced skills in the hunt seat discipline. In time, I developed a good foundation and was allowed to ride and show a couple of her multinational champions at local and regional levels in Washington State. People involved with the Arabian hunter jumper circuit may well remember the horses I

< 32 >

rode: With Regard and Barankwa, two geldings who earned many titles in the hunter world in the late 1970s through the mid-1980s. I realize now learning to jump on horses of that caliber was indeed a rare and unusual opportunity, and I feel so fortunate to have had it—it gave me something to look forward to and excel at.

Looking back, I believe having that experience in my teen years was a crucial turning point for me. All my family members struggled to deal with the trauma that happened to us. Some of them coped in ways that were not the best lifestyle choices.

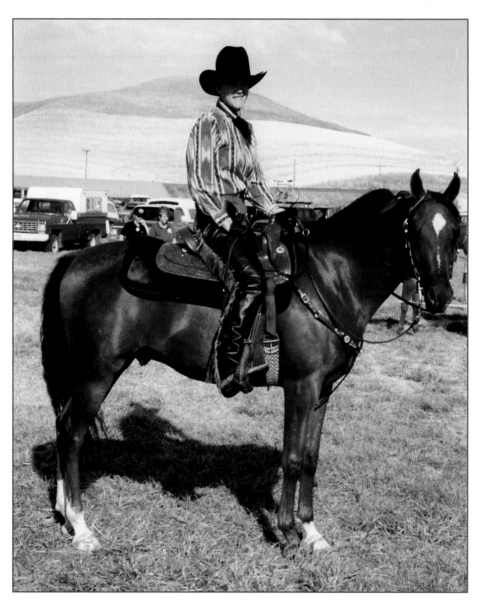

Sue and Shad

I feel I could very easily have gone in a less than positive direction had I not pursued horsemanship. In short, my brother's early gift started me on the road to emotional recovery. Starting with the horses of my youth, I learned life skills like confidence, leadership, and poise. I eventually got over my extreme shyness and a lot of other insecurities. My bad dreams went away, and I did very well in school.

During college and for a year or so after I was married, I did not have a horse to ride. I felt incomplete and stressed out. I started looking for a horse and found a gorgeous red dun mare. I brought her home and immediately felt more grounded and more like myself. Unfortunately, she developed an irreversible lameness problem and I had to sell her. After this setback, I called Chris, a friend of mine who was also a horse trainer, and asked him to look for a horse I could lease. He suggested we look at an Arabian gelding he had started but was now just sitting in his owner's pasture. Shadrac had been a bottle baby, hand raised by a dear woman who didn't ride.

Before we got to her house, Chris said, "Now Shad is Darlene's baby, so just let me talk to her first to see if she's open to letting him go across the state." After a tryout period, Darlene agreed to the lease. Then an awesome, unexplainable thing happened. When Darlene and Chris pulled up to my barn with Shad in the trailer, Darlene got out and said, "I've been in this barn before. But there used to be saddles hanging from the ceiling." I felt my stomach flip a little as I explained I had recently removed three

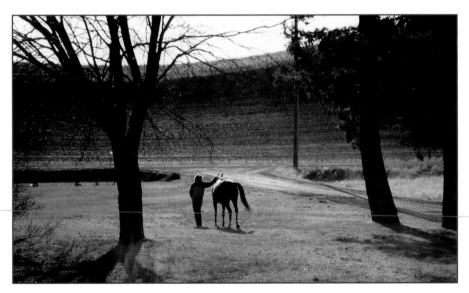

Sue walking Shad

or four saddles that had hung from the old barn's rafters for years. Yet we both knew she had never stepped foot on our property before that day. We took it as a sign that she made the right decision, and Shad was supposed to become my horse.

That was more than twenty years ago. The lease turned into a gift of ownership, and Darlene has since passed away. Shad has been with me all these years. He has helped both of my daughters learn to ride and is still my favorite, special companion even though I have another riding horse now.

It's been a long journey, and I still have some scars, but I think horses came into my life at a critical time and perhaps were divinely provided. These days, I'm part of a unique riding program that emphasizes training the whole horse physically, mentally, and emotionally through stress and recovery. We find these principles also apply to people like me who have suffered emotional stress but through horses are able to find a path toward mental, physical, and spiritual recovery. By sharing my story, I hope to illustrate to others how a lifelong relationship with horses can be more rewarding than any medicine a doctor could prescribe.

About Sue

Sue McMurray learned to ride seated behind a childhood friend on the back of Babe, an old Palomino mare. Graduating to the "driver's seat" sparked a lifelong passion for horsemanship. Sue now lives in Pullman, Washington, with her husband and two daughters. She enjoys training and showing her AQHA gelding, Doc's Driftin' Fox (Mac), in local open shows.

DOC, SMOKEY, OR BABE

— Terry Armstrong —

"When let go, horses will almost always find

their way back home to the barn."

Ray Armstrong was born in 1908 in southern Idaho to an old-school rancher and horseman. Riding horses was just a way of life for young Ray, and he never gave much thought to the hours he spent in the saddle growing up, even though it had a significant impact on his fitness, independence, and trail savvy, which would come back to serve him in his later years. As a hard-working ranch youth, Ray learned enough about horses and ranching to guide him through life, enabling him to become independent at a very young age.

Ray's father was a mean old rancher, according to his grandson, Terry. One day when Ray was only thirteen or fourteen years old, he finally had enough of his father and the strict ranch way of life and took off on his own, thinking of freedom and adventure. At that point in his life, Ray did not even know how to read. As a matter of fact, he had never attended school. He was able to teach himself to read a few words—just enough to get by on his own. That was the only way he—amazingly—managed to manipulate his way through the tests required for employment by the U.S. Forest Service when he was seventeen years old.

"My father didn't remember ever going to school, but somehow he managed to pass that test," said Ray's son, Terry. Although a minor, Ray, having grown up on a ranch, knew the ins and outs of horseback riding and cattle driving, so he managed well enough with the forest service. The high mountain plateaus and rugged ravines of the southern Idaho and northern Nevada country were no challenge to Ray—until one early spring blizzard, when he found himself trapped in the wilderness with no clue how to find his way back home.

It was in the spring of 1925, and young Ray was fulfilling his duties as a U.S. Forest Service employee in Nevada. Back then, ranchers free-ranged their cattle; whenever disputes arose over cattle grazing on the wrong ridge, it was the job of the forest service employees to check it out and drive the cattle back to their own allotted land. It was one of the jobs that Ray didn't really enjoy anyway, but this particular day was one he never forgot. If not for his trusty horse, he's certain he wouldn't have survived to tell the story to his children and grandchildren.

Ray had been assigned to the Pole Creek Ranger Station near Elko, Nevada, which was part of the Jarbidge Ranger District that was designated in the 1980s as a wilderness area. Now more than 113,000 acres, the area is part of the Humboldt-Toiyabe National Forest—the only national forest in Nevada and the largest in the United States. The remote, rugged area was as beautiful as it was mysterious. Just as the slopes and plateaus began to sprout with columbine, geranium, lupine, and mule ears, Ray received an assignment to go up and check on some cattle that had strayed from their designated area.

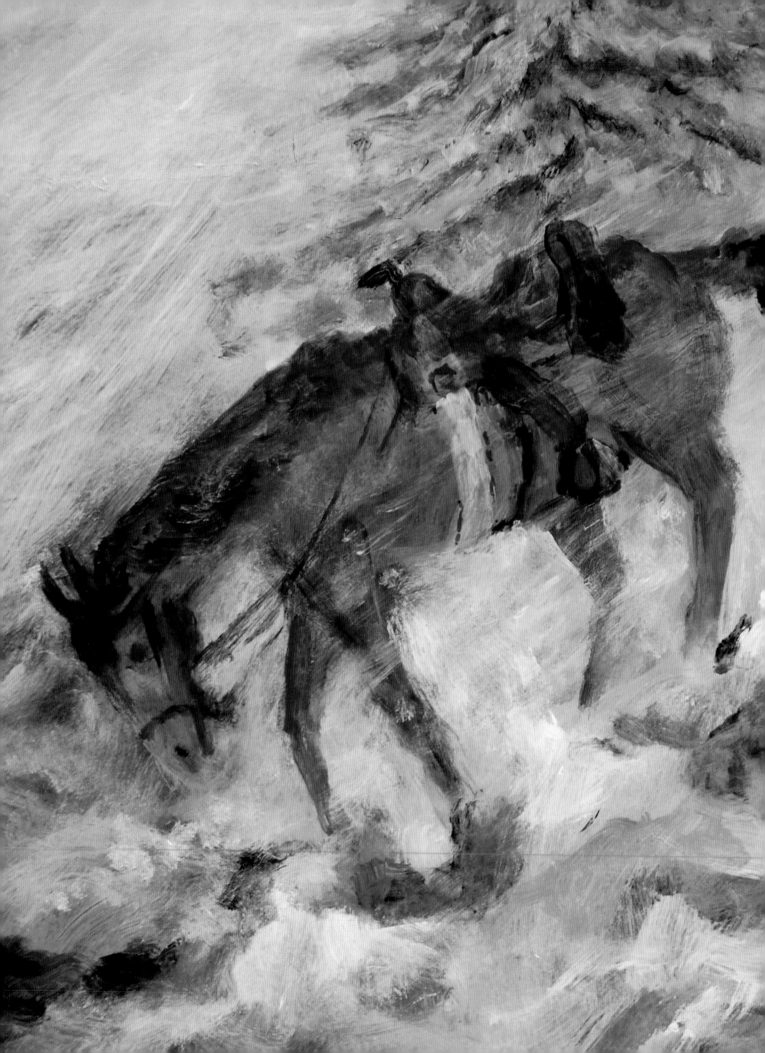

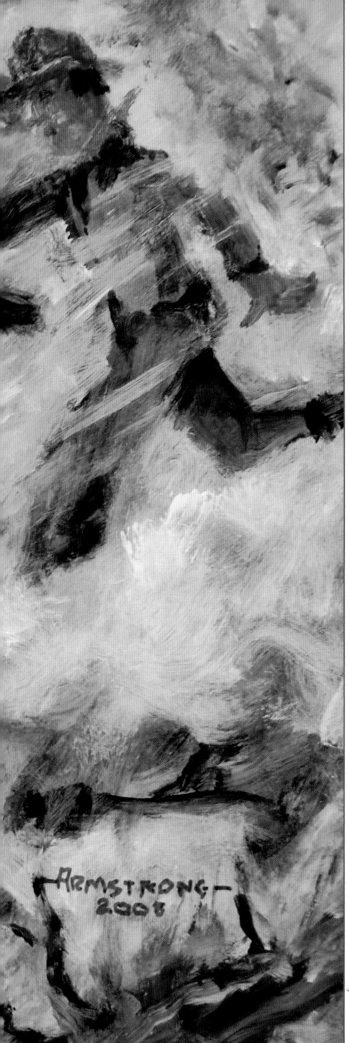

The early morning was cool as Ray set out from Pole Creek Ranger Station, intent on finding and rounding up the stray cattle. Mounted on his trusty horse Smokey, Doc, or Babe—son Terry can't recall—Ray made his way into the high desert country, unprepared for what he was about to encounter.

"It is really, really rugged territory," said Terry. "Very high plateau country and very steep trails, and Dad says he rode up there to check on these cattle, when it suddenly started to rain really hard." Rain on dust quickly turns to slick mud, making steep slopes treacherous for any animal, including Ray's horse. But matters quickly turned worse when the rain turned to snow and the wind kicked up. Before he knew it or could do anything about it, Ray was in the middle of a spring blizzard whiteout.

"The trail got real slippery," said Terry. "And then when it started to snow, he couldn't see a thing. The trail was gone and he had no idea how to get back to the ranger station. Here he was in this rugged, isolated territory all alone. In spite of all his experience, he said he was pretty scared."

In no time at all, Ray became disoriented. On instinct, he dismounted and left

◄ Terry Armstrong's rendition of his father

his horse, searching for the trail that led back down to the ranger station, which was now covered with snow. But his attempts failed. Still unable to see or find the trail, he made his way back to his horse—which had stayed put where Ray left him—deciding it would be best to stay close to something warm.

As he stood beneath a pine tree that shielded him from the driving snowfall, Ray suddenly recalled something about horses he'd known his entire life—one good thing his father had taught him that stuck. When let go, horses will almost always find their way back home to the barn. With that, Ray threw the horse's reins over its back, stepped behind the horse, wrapped its tail around his hands, and held on with all his strength. Then he closed his eyes and let the horse take over.

Ray's horse began its descent down the mountain, unaffected by the human appendage that stumbled and slipped along behind. Head down in the blinding snowstorm, the horse carefully guided Ray back to safety.

"Dad was never so glad to get back home," said Terry. "As tough as he was, this experience humbled him and made him realize what a great horse he had."

Because of his horse's natural instincts, Ray lived to tell the story over and over to his children and grandchildren. In 2008, he would have been 100 years old. Terry, an accomplished educator and talented painter, loves retelling cowboy stories of his father and grandfather.

Ray Armstrong went on to become a successful cattleman and accomplished horseman, but the story of the day his horse saved his life was rarely far from his memory. Although he rode many horses throughout his life, he always remembered fondly that one who literally pulled him to safety.

BACARDI 151

— *Sherriey Miller* —

"My horses are my friends, my confidants, my loves, my saviors. Even today, they are my reason for living, my reason for getting up and going to work—my sanity."

As a little girl, Sherriey Miller found comfort, love, and peace in horse books from the school library, mostly from the Grossit & Dunlap *Famous Horse Stories* series and books by Walter Farley and Marguerite Henry. Living in a family with an abusive and dominant mother, Sherriey thought of her fantasy horses as lifesavers. They helped her get through her early years, but also instilled within her a deep desire to own a real, flesh-and-blood horse some day.

Sherriey left home when she was eighteen with the first man who paid her any attention. He bought her a horse, which turned out to be a great comfort to her when her relationship with the man went south. "I'd hide and cry into my horse's mane, where I felt loved and safe," said Sherriey. Before long, the man proved to be abusive as well, and again Sherriey ran away.

Trying to find some comfort and establish roots, Sherriey eventually started a horse herd of her own. Of them, one gelding stands out above the rest. He was a little 14-hand blue roan Appaloosa with spots named Bacardi 151.

Bacardi was a great trail horse that Sherriey took a fondness to. The two of them formed a deep kinship. "He was my watch dog," said Sherriey. "If I wasn't out there and someone tried to enter the pasture, he'd lay his ears and charge at a full gallop. Believe me, they'd be running full speed to escape Bacardi!"

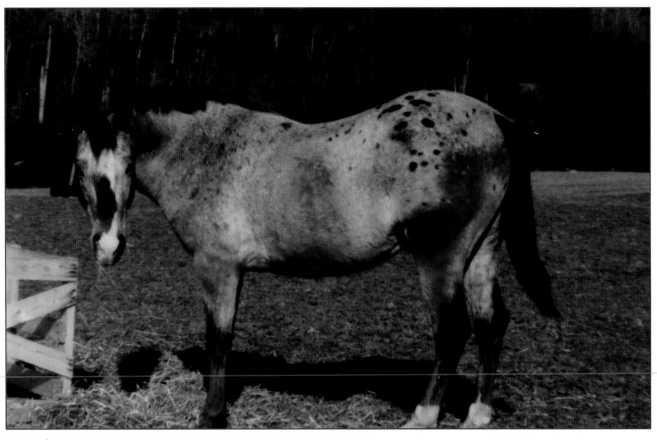

Bacardi 151 in 1984

During this time, a friend of Sherriey had a little dark brown grade mare named Lena who was pastured with Bacardi. When it came to feeding time, Lena would turn wicked and unpredictable. Sherriey tried to keep a close watch on Lena and stay clear of her as much as possible. But she wasn't always successful.

"One evening at chore time, I was bringing out the hay and had to go past Lena to get to the feeder," said Sherriey. "She reached to grab the hay from me, and I turned so she couldn't get at it. That really made her angry!"

Sherriey immediately knew she was in danger, and she tried to move out of the way quickly. But Lena wheeled and let both feet fly, hitting Sherriey in the side and leg. Sherriey fell to the ground with a broken leg. As she lay there trying to decide what to do, she was horrified at what she saw next. Lena had turned and was coming after her.

"I couldn't get up because my leg was broken, so I rolled toward the fence to get away from her. Still, Lena came at me with her hooves and her bared teeth, determined to do me in. I screamed for help and curled into the fetal position, figuring I was going to get trampled."

Bacardi heard his owner's scream. He was off on the other side of the barn, and when he heard the scream, he came running to see what was wrong. "When he saw what was happening, in a split second he was straddling over the top of me with his ears pinned at Lena—warning her not to come a step closer. I opened my eyes to see the belly of a horse over me, protecting me."

After Lena backed off, Bacardi then turned and went over to eat like nothing ever happened. "I will never forget that little horse," said Sherriey. "I truly believe he saved my life."

But that wasn't the end of Bacardi's life-saving days. He had proven to be rock solid with children, so Sherriey eventually sold him to a young girl as a trail horse. One day his new owner was trail riding with a girlfriend, when suddenly the girlfriend was thrown from her horse into a deep swale. The girl struggled but couldn't get out.

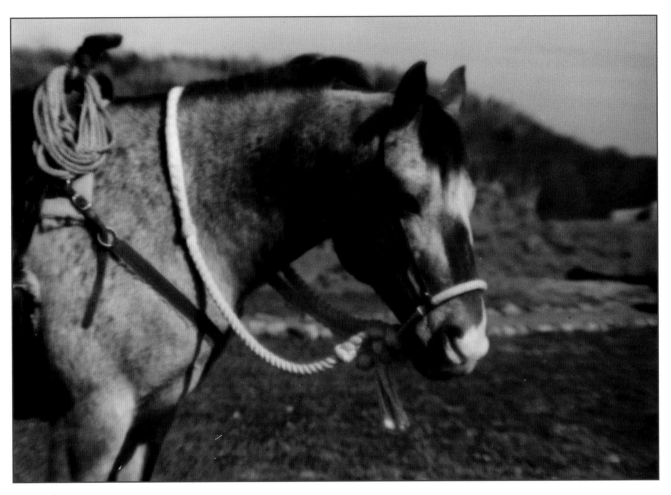

Bacardi 151 in 1984

Bacardi's new owner got off him and instructed him to go down into the rocky pit while her friend called to him. He knew exactly what he was supposed to do. He carefully slid down into the pit and stood quietly while the injured girl mounted him. After several attempts to get out of the steep swale, he finally carried her to safety.

"So I guess he saved her, too," said Sherriey. "Bacardi was a wonderful friend. My horses are my friends, my confidants, my loves, and my saviors. Even today, they are my reason for living, my reason for getting up and going to work, my sanity. I couldn't, wouldn't, exist or be who I am without them. They are my universe and my life. I love them as a mother loves a child. They aren't just horses—they are my life."

THERAPY

—— Celia Working ——

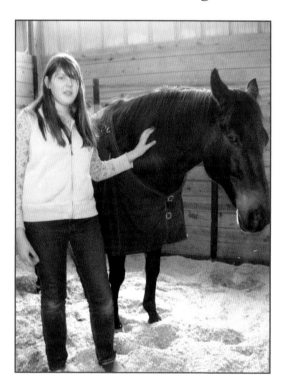

Here we go—a new day begins

And I get ready to collect my wins.

When I started working at TRC,

Little did I know, the therapy would be for me.

For it's not just the ones who ride

Who leave here with a sense of pride.

It's a feeling I would have never guessed—

It goes to show how much I'm blessed.

For these horses don't see "student" or "staff"

They just see people who need a good laugh.

We all need a boost, in confidence or spirit,

And all of these horses—well, they want to hear it!

Yes, when I started at TRC,

Little did I know, the therapy would be for me.

About Celia

Celia is a volunteer at Fieldstone Farm Therapeutic Riding Center in Chagrin Falls, Ohio.

CARNIVAL: THE KING THAT SAVED MY LIFE

—— Ryan Towne ——

"My goal is to someday leave my wheelchair and walk again.

I really long to get my life back."

Some people might call life in a wheelchair a "life," but not me. I've been active my entire life, so when an automobile accident left me wheelchair-bound, I wasn't sure I'd ever really "live" again. That is, until Carnival King came into my life—a huge English Thoroughbred who gave me back mobility and, most of all, hope.

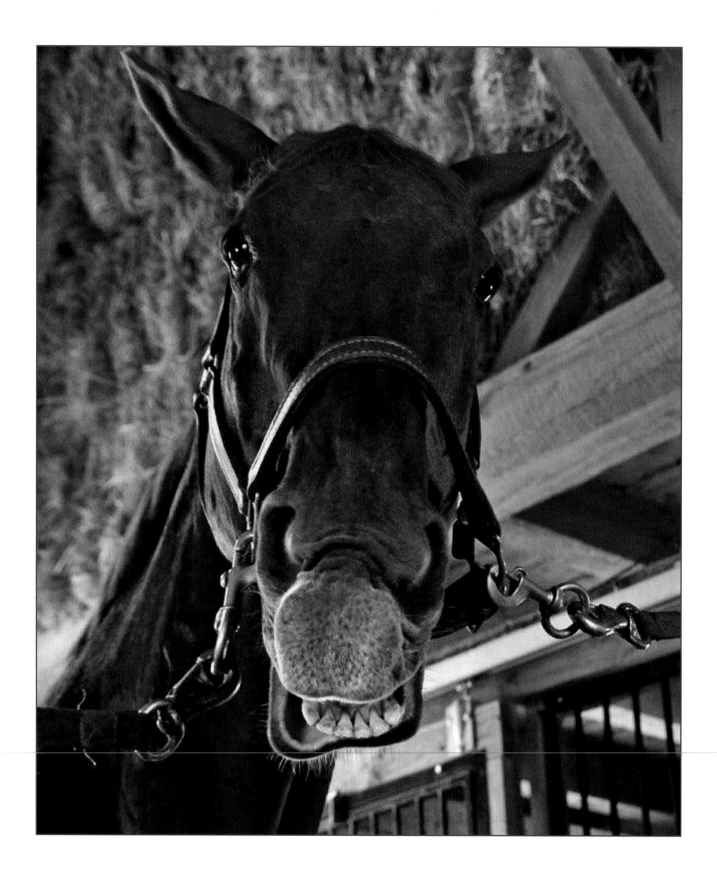

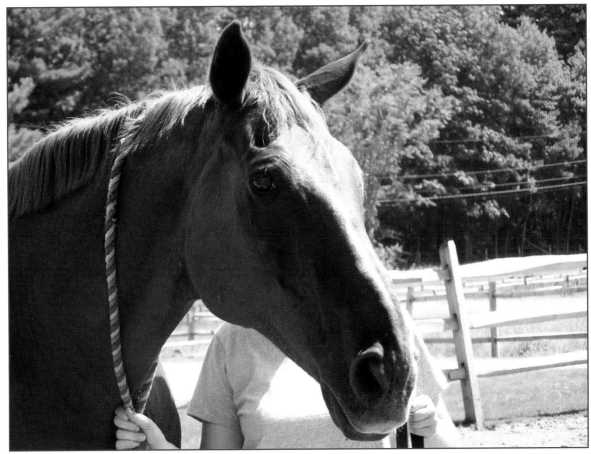

Carnival King

I was born in 1975, the second of two children and the first boy to Robert and Gerry Towne. I have an older sister, Amy, who has two boys, Mat and Jacob, and a newborn girl, Heather.

I was mischievous and a daredevil from the start—from my high school days as an ice hockey player to snowboarding on the slopes of Sunday River in Maine. I also enjoyed deep-sea diving and volunteered for the Kennebunk Fire Department. When it came to work, the more dangerous the better. I worked as an explosive technician assistant prior to becoming a cellular communications installer, climbing towers up to 1,800 feet high. Life for me was all about being on the go and pushing the limits.

◄ Carnival had a sense of humor

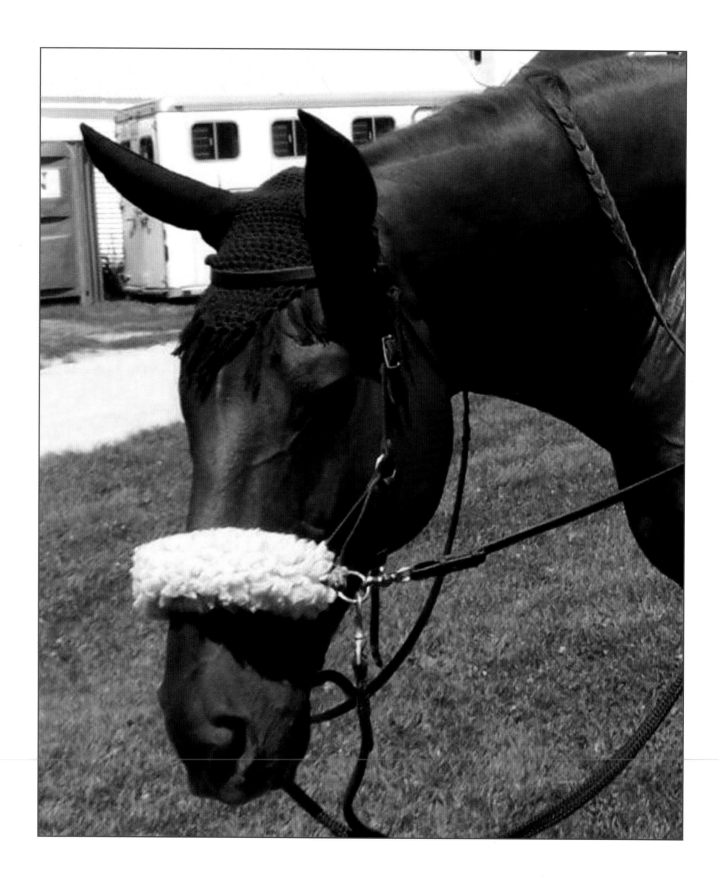

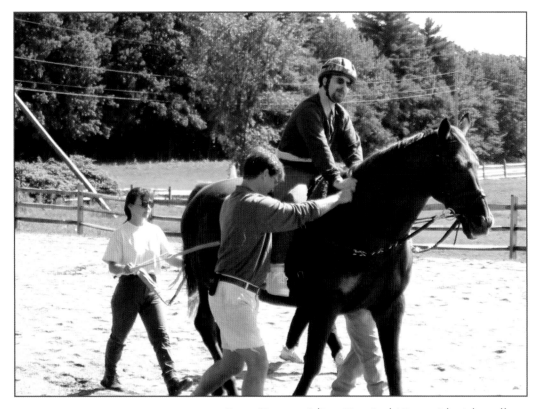

Ryan Towne riding Carnival King with sidewalkers

It's hard to look back on those days before the accident, when life was carefree and easy—before my life was plagued with survival. But I prefer to look forward now because I've been given a second chance. Let me tell you my story.

On a fall evening in October 2000, when I was twenty-five years old, I was driving my buddies home from an evening out. I was the designated driver. I had a 1994 full-size Stepside Chevy with a three-inch body lift kit to allow for four 33-inch Thornbird tires. (Did I say that I was very much into vehicles back then?) On the way home, I was blinded by a bright light and lost control of my truck on a sharp curve. The truck left the road and rolled over. I was thrown out. I wasn't wearing my seatbelt.

The pickup rolled over my head, causing severe brain injury. I was airlifted to Maine Medical Center in Portland, Maine, in critical condition. Time was of the essence. Luckily, my buddies suffered just minor injuries.

◄ Carnival King

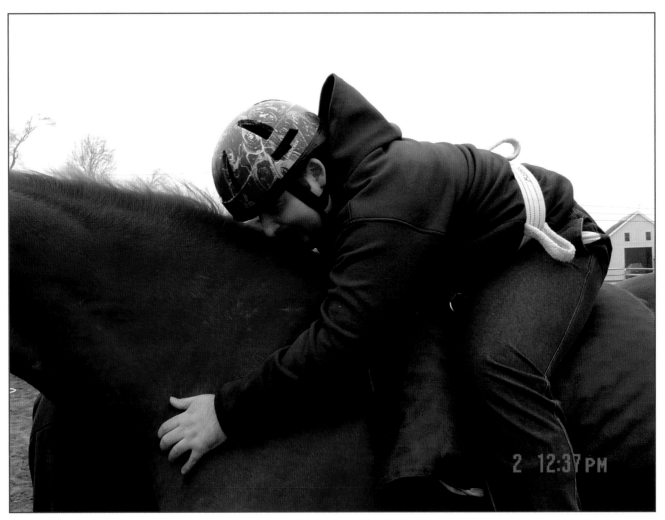

Ryan Towne on Carnival King

My dad was on a ship check in San Diego, California at the time and rushed home to be by my side. But before he arrived, Mom was there to make some very hard decisions on her own. She chose to give me a chance at life by agreeing to surgery to remove a blood clot that had formed at the base of my brain. It was a very risky operation. There were no guarantees I would live after the clot was removed. It was a miracle I survived.

I was in a coma for four months. Between hospitals and a rehabilitation facility, I didn't come home for a full year. Even though my mind is now clear, the brain injury has affected my mobility and my speech. I am in a wheelchair. My goal is to someday leave my wheelchair and walk again. I really long to get my life back.

My road to recovery, while it is still not complete, began when I was introduced to hippotherapy. I first met Sue Grant (a.k.a Helga) in May 2002 at Equest Therapeutic Riding Center at Spring Creek Farm in Lyman, Maine—a therapeutic horseback riding facility. Little did I know the positive influence she and the entire staff would have on me and my family, not to mention the horse who became my best friend and who showed me deep compassion—an English Thoroughbred named Carnival King. On Carnival, I didn't feel handicapped anymore—I felt free.

Freedom: no walls closing in on me, fresh air, a chance to be outside, pleasant memories of my Bumpa (grandfather) on his farm, and, most of all, *hope*. These were some of my feelings when I was on Carnival's back.

Carnival King came to Equest after retiring from a long, competitive career in the showing, hunting, and eventing world. Foaled in Ireland and shown in England for the first half of his life, he accumulated numerous Hunter and Working Hunter Championships, culminating in winning the Middleweight Hunter of the Year title at the Horse of the Year show held in London in 1989. His lineage boasts of royalty and more fame, with a sire who was owned by the Queen, and a brother—Duneight Carnival—who competed at the Barcelona Olympics. Carnival's grandsire, Crepello, won the English Derby in 1957.

Carnival King was purchased in 1990 by a British woman living in the United States, who continued to show him in eventing and dressage competitions until he was nineteen years old. In 2000, his owner decided to retire Carnival, but she knew that being "turned out to pasture" was not the right fit for him, so she donated him to the Equest Therapeutic Riding Center to be a therapy horse for handicapped, aspiring equestrians like myself. Forever a professional when it comes to his work, with his large stature but gentle and noble qualities, Carnival proudly lived out his twilight years carrying Equest's disabled riders to new heights (literally!).

Carnival was a beautiful chestnut-colored horse. In some ways he was like a pet, and yet he was so much more. He was loyal. He made me feel safe and secure and, more than anything else, he gave me freedom. When I was on his back, I didn't have a worry in the world. I loved that horse.

When I was on Carnival King's back, I felt like I was *someone* again. It was the one place I could go where I wasn't handicapped any longer! Where I didn't have to be in this chair, yet I could still get around. He took me places my legs and wheelchair couldn't.

Carnival King would put himself under me when I started to get tired and lean to one side. And he would stop when he sensed that I had a problem. When I stretched while on his back, he didn't get spooked when I shifted my weight or had a muscle spasm. He always stayed calm, so I always felt safe on him. Riding Carnival King felt more like recreation than therapy.

The rhythmic motion of horseback riding has stimulated my pelvis and trunk, making me stronger. When I started riding I could walk with assistance approximately twenty-five feet. After four months of riding, that increased to more than 300 feet with minimal assistance. Riding has helped me hold up my head and chest, which allows me to talk more freely and more frequently than I have in the past. Now that I'm controlling the horse on my own, sidewalkers are there only to cushion my fall. But I have no intention of falling.

I start each session by standing and grooming my horse. I like this part of the session because it gives me a chance to stand and stretch before I ride. And I think Carnival liked it best because it was my way of showing him how much I appreciated and loved him.

Next I go to the indoor ring so the staff can lift me onto the horse using the electric lift. This makes it easier on my horse and me, and I don't waste any more energy before I ride. Now all the work begins. Sidewalkers bring me out to the center of the ring to get me centered on my horse's back.

I am also graduating to a saddle! Previously I was using a fleece blanket on top with a surcingle to hold onto. A surcingle is a leather strap with a metal handle. Now that I'll be using a saddle—giddy-up—no more rawhide!

I continue to do therapeutic horseback riding and continue to work toward my goal of leaving my wheelchair behind. My hope is that therapeutic horseback riding will help me reach that goal someday. It's been a long, hard road back, but thanks to Carnival, I'm on my way.

Carnival passed away when he was twenty-seven years old. He will be missed by many, but especially by me. I couldn't have asked for a better horse or for a better first experience. I don't know what I would have done without him.

My family has stood by me through this difficult ordeal. My father, Bob Towne, is often one of my sidewalkers at Equest.

"None of us knew the depth of Ryan's feelings when riding until he told his story," said Bob. "To know what my son feels when riding is worth more than anyone can possibly imagine."

FRECKLES AND TOM

— Liz Kinkaid —

"My heart was pounding. Tom had heard me say to let go of the horn and he did—but one of his feet slid through the stirrup and now he hung upside down."

It was a big moment in my life when my young son, nearly seven years old, decided he wanted to go riding with his mom. I had always hoped that one of my three children would want to ride horses and have the passion for them that I did. I was smiling from ear to ear. I wanted to stop traffic and knock on doors: "See? Will ya look at that? Just look at *my boy* on that horse!"

Tom sat proudly on a rather tall, spotted gelding; a chestnut leopard Appaloosa. His little legs could barely reach the stirrups on the adult Western saddle, and the seat had room for at least two more riders. He sat with one very little hand on the horn and the reins in his other hand, holding them just like I had shown him before we left the house for our mini-trail ride around the neighborhood. His big blue eyes were filled with thoughts of our adventure, and his golden locks played in the gusty breezes that were swirling about that day.

Freckles, the leopard gelding, was careful in his movements, walking at a steady pace and stopping when the reins commanded him to. My son was absolutely amazed at the power he had over this gigantic, gentle beast. The longer we rode, the more confident I could see my son become. We tried a trot, and Tom squealed with laughter. It wasn't long before he began to lose his seat, but the horse instinctively slowed to a walk and then stopped completely for Tom to regain his balance. I was laughing too, so thrilled to be able to experience the joy of my son's first big ride outside of our own small pasture!

The beautiful young mare that I rode, a three-year-old, was reacting to every little leaf that the wind managed to blow her way, snorting and sometimes quickly sidestepping in an attempt to escape possible harm from the autumn leaves. She was learning and getting better with every ride, but she still had a way to go before she was calm. She was a beautiful black mare with a large blanket over her rump with baseball-sized black spots scattered throughout. She was a stunning creature to behold.

There was a wonderful field across the street from our house that had been cleared by our neighbors, who had given us permission to ride there anytime. That would be our way home—around the back of our neighbor's house through the field and then across the street to our barn. Years ago when the neighbors had built their home, they had a pond dug and stocked with fish. It was a very tranquil spot; we often visited with old bread to feed to the ducks that lived there. The owners had also put in a fountain to help aerate the pond.

As we approached the field, Tom wanted to go over to look at the water. He urged the gelding forward and pushed him into a very slow trot, with his head low and the reins loose. I trotted up beside him, almost sad that our ride was coming to an end.

As we stood there horse by horse staring at the ducks paddling in the water, we started to hear sputtering and crackling. My mare began nervously moving, and as I tried to control her, I looked about trying to figure out where the noise was coming from. Then the explosion of water happened. The fountain went off like a geyser! My mare reared straight up, and I almost came out of the saddle. Tom screamed. Freckles stood his ground. When my mare came down she bolted—and that was when the Freckles lost his cool and also bolted, with Tom screaming in terror on his back. He was not an experienced enough rider to instinctively gather the reins at the sign of trouble. As a matter of fact, he had dropped his reins.

I was able to gather up my reins and stop the mare. Freckles, however, ran, and Tom was tossed helplessly about in the saddle.

"*Hold on!*" I screeched. "*Hold onto the horn!*" With my reins pulled tight and my mare circling and jumping about, I tried to keep my eyes on the runaway pair, trying to yell encouragement to my small son. The big horse was running back to the barn and heading right for the street in the process. Tom was screaming, scared to death. With the mare under some control, I took off after the uncontrolled gelding. I couldn't take my eyes off the two of them. That was my child on the back of that horse—my baby. My mind was whirling in a thousand different directions, and I don't remember breathing at all.

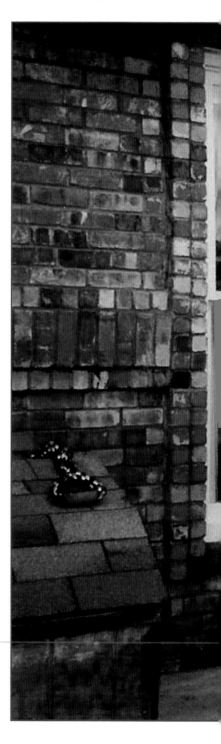

Soon after I started out after the two of them, Tom slipped to the side of the saddle. His weight was out of the seat; he was gripping the horn with every bit of strength that he had, crying for help and screaming as he hung off the side of the horse.

Then like magic, Freckles just stopped. Tom's legs dangled and he struggled to find a stirrup. "Just let go of the horn!" I screamed, thinking he could just slip to the ground unharmed. "Let go!" Fearing if I ran up to them I would start the gelding running again, I stopped my mare and tried to talk to Tom from a distance. Freckles was nervously picking up his front feet,

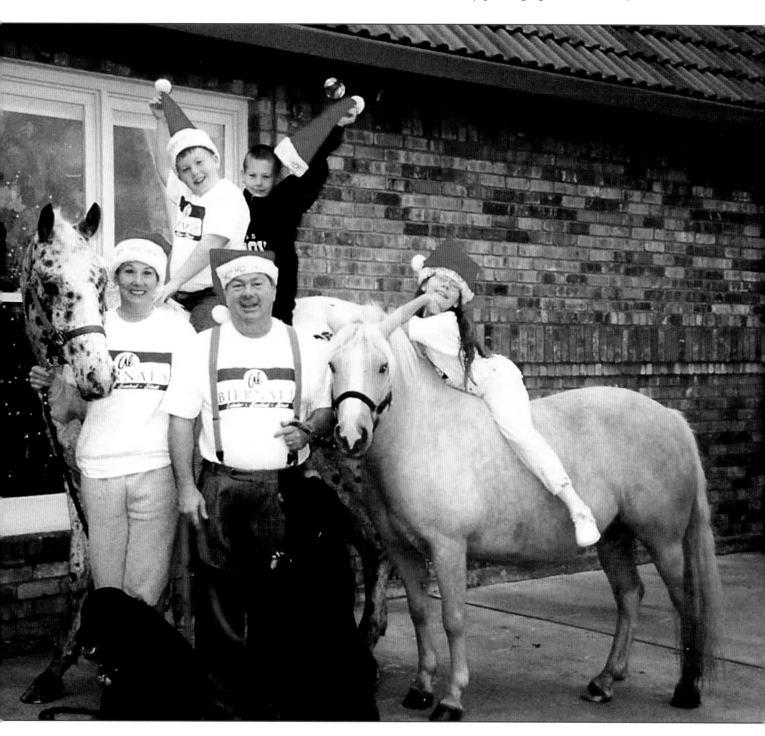

walking in place. Up, down, up, down … like he was getting ready to race. My heart was pounding. Tom had heard me say to let go of the horn, and he finally did—but one of his feet had slid through the stirrup and now he hung upside down.

"O Dear God, *no!*" I said out loud, "*Dear God, no!*" If that horse took off my baby could die. I went numb.

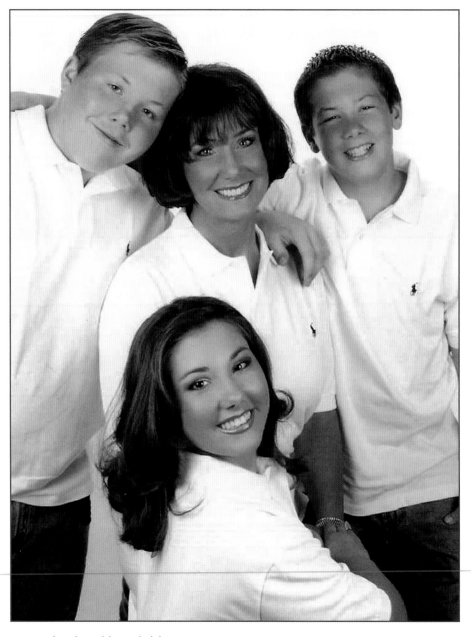

Liz Kinkaid and her children

Freckles anxiously watched Tom hanging from the stirrup, and he tossed his head and flung the reins up in the air. He was fighting his instincts with all his might. But he stood still. I must have screamed "Kick your foot loose!" a thousand times, over and over and over and over again. And then, finally, Tom did it. He kicked his foot loose. It was like someone had taken a pair of scissors and separated the boy from his trap. When he plopped to the ground, the gelding galloped off, following the street, which opened out to a very busy intersection. I knew in my heart he would be killed, but my main concern was for my little boy, who lay crying hysterically on the pavement.

My young son—scared to death—was alive. I rode up and got off my mare. I had to hold her tightly as she too was dancing about and still silly from all the confusion. I leaned over and picked up my little boy and held him to me tightly. We were both crying.

"Thank you!" I whispered to God. My mind started to function again, and I thought to ask Tom if he was OK.

"I was (*sniff*) so (*sniff, sniff*) scared, Mom!" he said between gulps of air.

"Oh, honey, you were so brave!" I told him. "I am so proud of you! I am so sorry that happened!" My own throat was so tight I could barely breathe.

Tom raised his head up to look around and then pointed his finger and said, "Look!"

I turned to look where he was pointing. There, walking back toward us, with his reins dragging, was Freckles. It then occurred to me that he had stopped when Tom had left the seat of the saddle. Had he been a calf-roping horse? Had he been trained to know that when one left the seat of the saddle he must stop? How did he know to do what he did? What I *did* know was this: The big Appaloosa gelding had stayed true to his training and had literally saved the life of my child. Although his natural instincts were to run with fear, when Tom's life was in danger, Freckles literally protected him.

I couldn't sleep that night thinking of what could have happened if the horse had taken off again when my son's foot hung in the stirrup. I shudder even today thinking about what could have been.

Little Tom never got back on another horse, but that's okay. He never realized how lucky he was to be on that particular horse that day. Dear sweet Freckles was sold to a family that had grandchildren riding him, and they called once to tell me he is the most gentle horse; so kind with the children. I smiled and thought to myself, *You don't even know.*

About Liz

Liz Kincaid lives in Texas and has three children: Ashley, T. K., and Warren. They are her whole world. When the kids are off with their friends or busy with school activities, Liz can be found at her barn working with her beautiful Appaloosas or spoiling Bay Bars Silver, her Appaloosa hero and inspiration.

VALENTINO'S STORY

—— *Lisa Wysocky* ——

"I had no clue what was happening, but thank goodness I knew

enough to realize that a horse is smarter than a human."

Afew years ago, I found myself holding my breath in the center of Miller
Coliseum on the campus of Middle Tennessee State University as I prepared to longe
a then four-year-old Tennessee Walking Horse-large pony cross. The horse, Valentino,
and I were part of a therapeutic riding demonstration at the Volunteer Horse Fair,
Tennessee's annual statewide horse expo, and there were several thousand people in
the audience as I played out the longe line.

The reason I was holding my breath was because this wasn't just any horse, and this wasn't just any longeing session. This was a horse who had been abandoned as a yearling; his human family had moved away and left him alone in a field to fend for himself. When various neighbors remembered, or had the money, they would throw this little black horse some hay. After a year or so, Horse Haven of Tennessee, an equine rescue organization in the Knoxville area, stepped in and rescued him. He came to a therapeutic riding program in Middle Tennessee a few months later—having been fed, wormed, and gelded—after three sessions as a demonstration horse for equine clinician Craig Cameron at that year's Tennessee Horse Fair. At the time of his arrival, Valentino was not halter broke, did not tie, and, due to his prolonged isolation as a youngster, had no idea how to relate to people, much less other horses.

The first day Valentino arrived at his new home, he became so agitated he flew around his pasture at a full gallop and eventually jumped a four-rail fence. It took me several weeks to get him to tie without the danger of him hurting himself or the people around him, and for most of the first year, everything I introduced, he fought. But I knew that he fought out of fear and uncertainty, not out of aggressiveness. Remember, this is a horse who essentially grew up on the equivalent of a desert island and was then drop shipped into a barn that was as busy as the middle of New York City. Every new experience was quite overwhelming to him.

As I worked with Valentino (so named because even though he is a gelding, he does like the ladies), I realized how thoughtful and intelligent he was. Although untrained, at 14.2 hands, Valentino was the perfect size for many therapeutic program needs. He also had very rhythmic and cadenced gaits at the walk and trot, which is very important in therapeutic riding. Plus, he was smart and starved for affection, so the odds were that eventually he could be a valuable addition to the therapeutic riding community.

So here Valentino and I were a year later, in the center of the coliseum, ready to show the world how this ribby, untrained, unsocialized youngster went from a frightened loner to a trusting companion in less than a year.

Earlier I said this wasn't just any longeing session. And it was not. It was a demonstration to show how Valentino was desensitized and, in the process, learned to

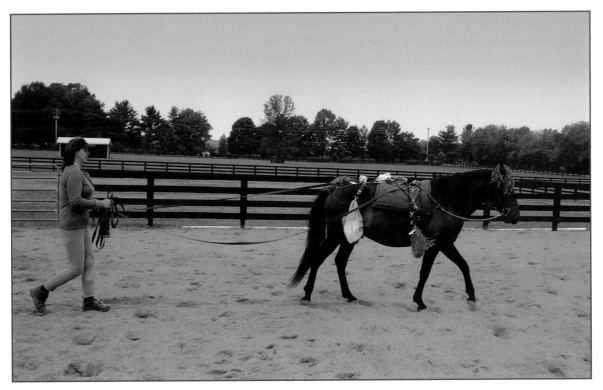

Lisa Wysocky drives Valentino

trust both himself and people. In addition to a halter and longe line, Valentino was wearing a longeing surcingle with ladder reins attached over his back and under his tail. Ladder reins are a piece of adaptive equipment sometimes used in therapeutic riding. Think of regular English reins with cross pieces, like rungs on a ladder, every six inches or so. Snapped to the surcingle and ladder reins were sleigh bells, a black plastic bag, rattles, a plastic grocery bag with a pie tin and plastic ball inside, two pompoms, a plastic milk jug with a few pebbles in it, a vinyl feed bag, and various cloth streamers. To top it off, around his neck he wore a multi-colored slinky and between his ears a colorful blue pompom. In short, Valentino looked like a junkman's truck and sounded like a one-horse band.

Of course, he didn't start out with all that equipment. We began by slowly introducing one piece, and when he was fully comfortable with that, we added another, and another. The goal of Valentino's desensitization was to accustom him to different groups of objects that encompassed various colors, sounds, and movement. Then, hopefully, when he encountered an unusual situation, he would fall back on his training, rather than react out of fear.

Valentino had been through so much of this training at home that this very extraordinary group of objects had become, to him, routine. The training also built his trust in his human partners and confidence in himself. But with the added stimulation of new surroundings, the echo of the loudspeaker, movement of people in the stands, and the wide-open space of the arena, would Valentino remember his training, or would he panic and try to flee? That's why I was holding my breath.

Remembering how important human physical demeanor is to the horse, I let out my breath, swallowed my doubt, presented confident body language, and played out the longe line with a command of "Valentino, walk on." For the next ten minutes Valentino quietly and confidently walked, trotted, cantered, reversed, and stopped on command, his head low, his ears flicking in my direction, as I explained the desensitization process to the audience.

I have been proud of many things in my life, but this little horse is close to the top of the list. He came a long way in a very short time, but this is not the end of Valentino's story. In fact, it is only the beginning. I mention it because what comes next shows that a little love, attention, and patience can actually save your life.

Early one evening, some time after I had come to know Valentino, I was leading him from the pasture into the barn. As soon as he set foot in the barn on this particular day, he stopped, and I knew something was wrong. During the time I had worked with him, we got to know each other very well, and he was a horse who was usually very eager to go wherever you asked. He is always up for a new adventure and, with his half Walking Horse heritage, takes long, confident strides. Now, he not only stopped, but he turned his left shoulder toward me and moved his rear end away from me. In essence, he was blocking my path into the barn.

Then Valentino did something even stranger. He ducked his head down and to the right and pinned his ears. I had no clue what was happening, but thank goodness I knew enough to realize that a horse is smarter than a human. I'm glad I understood that, because my hesitation might have saved my life. A few seconds later, a coyote walked out from an open stall. Valentino had known he was there, and he was using his body to block and protect me from the wild animal.

In the dim light in the barn I could see that the coyote was quite thin, and its hair coat was matted and mangy. And rather than growling, snarling, or showing other aggressive behavior, the animal swayed back and forth. But his eyes never left Valentino's. After what seemed like an eternity, the coyote turned and walked out the open door at the far end of the barn and disappeared into the tall grass in a field next to another pasture. He never looked back.

As soon as the animal left the barn, Valentino relaxed. His head came back up and he looked at me as if to say, "It's okay now, so let's get going." But I wasn't quite as sure as Valentino, so we stayed frozen to the spot until my heart stopped thumping in my chest and I could once again begin to breathe. The entire episode probably did not last thirty seconds, but it seemed like forever.

Several days later a dead coyote was found in the back part of the pasture, and I have no doubt it was the same animal that we encountered in the barn. The coyote had looked and acted ill, or maybe he was very old. In either case, I know Valentino saved me from walking into the path of a dangerous wild animal and possibly even saved my life.

I was close to Valentino before then, but I now look at him with renewed respect. We've spent many hours sharing bonding time, with me sitting on a pasture fence watching him graze or finding the spots where he loves to be scratched. He apparently likes me well enough to leave his friends, whinny, and come galloping up to me when I walk into the pasture.

We also spend time playing with his new passion—a Frisbee. He loves watching the Frisbee fly through the air, and then he purposefully walks to its landing spot and picks it up in his mouth. Although he looks to me for guidance, I have not yet gotten him to bring it back to me. When I do, maybe you will see us on *America's Funniest Home Videos*.

While Valentino is my buddy and my trusted equine companion, he still helps people with disabilities learn to ride. As a registered NARHA instructor, I have come to trust Valentino, as he is the first to let me know when a rider is slightly off balance or when the rider is uncomfortable with the task at hand. I can tell by Valentino's glance, the length of his stride, or the flick of his tail what I need to do to deliver the most effective riding lesson possible.

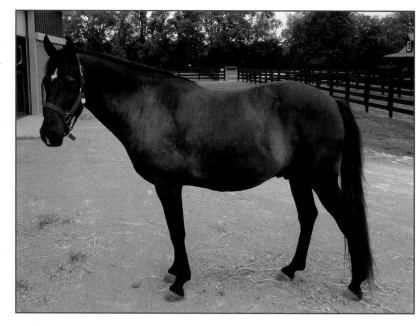

Valentino

At the time I am writing this, Valentino is just six years old. I look forward to spending many more years in his company, and I will never, ever forget that I owe my safety, and possibly my life, to this wonderful horse.

About Lisa

A nationally known equine clinician, Lisa Wysocky is a registered NARHA instructor and the author of *Horse Country: A Celebration of Country Music and the Love of Horses*, and *My Horse, My Partner: Teamwork on the Ground* (along with DVD). A former trainer of Appaloosa show horses, in 2007 Lisa was chosen by American Riding Instructors Association (ARIA) as one of the Top 50 riding instructors in the nation. In addition to her clinics and seminars, Lisa now trains horses for use in therapeutic riding programs and consults with NARHA programs across the country. She can be reached at www.LisaWysocky.com.

CALM IN THE PRESENCE OF DANGER

— *Terry Armstrong* —

. . . What he was about to encounter he still finds frightening and mysterious to this day.

The Taylor Ranch Wilderness Research Station is considered America's wildest classroom. It's not a recreation area, but a pristine, complex ecosystem set aside for research by the University of Idaho. The only access to this remote site is by hiking in thirty-two miles, or by small passenger plane, if your nerves can take landing on a short, grass airstrip in a deep mountain gorge.

The site is in the middle of the Frank Church River of No Return Wilderness Area, a sixty-five-acre block of untouched land surrounded by more than four million

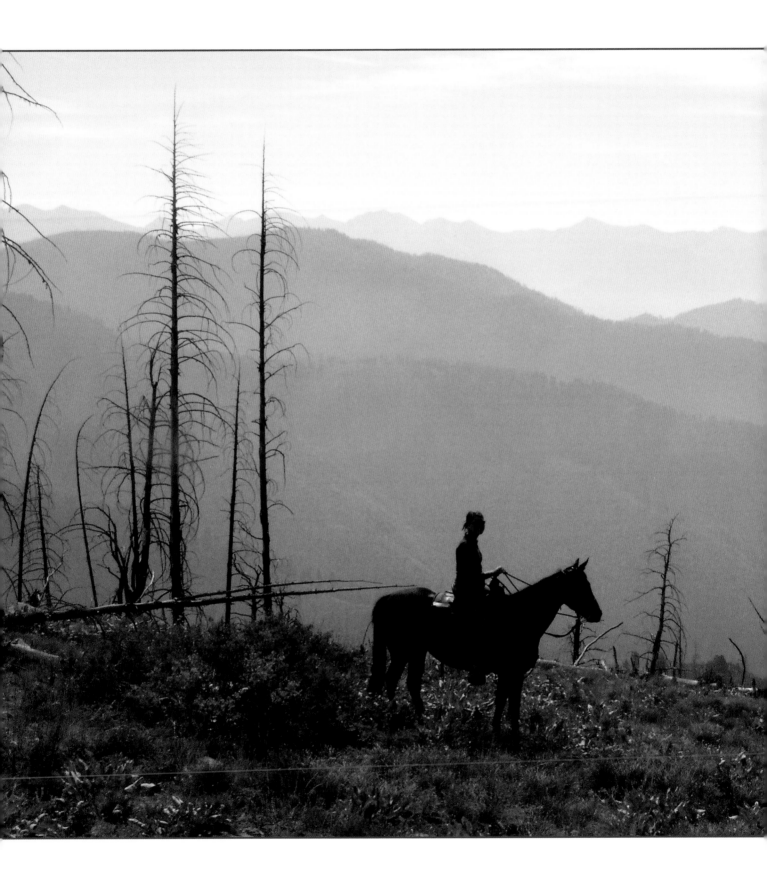

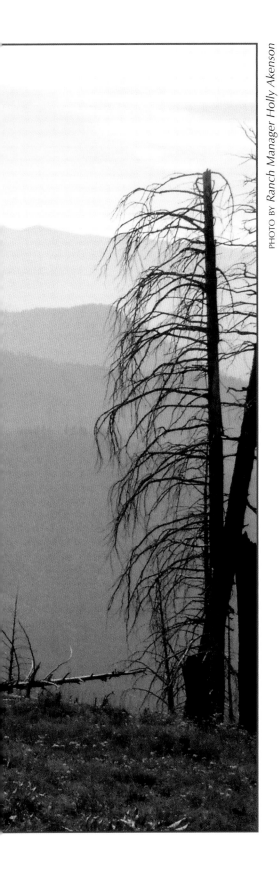

PHOTO BY *Ranch Manager Holly Akenson*

acres of even more wilderness. It is the largest block of wilderness in the lower forty-eight states.

Scientist Terry Armstrong, then the executive assistant to the president and coordinator of student services at the University of Idaho, set out for Taylor Ranch Wilderness Field Station in central Idaho in August of 1988 to have a look at the place, not realizing that he was about to have one of his most extraordinary life adventures. Nor was he aware that a stocky gray mare would become a major player in his next forty-eight hours.

Having grown up in southern Idaho, Terry knew he was flying into extreme wilderness. As a matter of fact, *extreme* spoke for all the characteristics of Taylor Ranch, from the weather to the geology to the animals and plants that inhabit the area—including rattlesnakes, mountain goats, and cougars.

The terrain of the area is deeply dissected and complex, creating a high level of biodiversity. A granite batholith covers much of the area and the climate varies dramatically due to the extremes in elevation and the rain shadow effect of high-elevation peaks. This varied climate change would have a major impact on Terry's time at the ranch. As a matter of fact, what he was about to encounter he still finds frightening and mysterious to this day.

Historically, studies at Taylor have focused on the relationships between wildlife and vegetation, wildlife

◄ Ellen Hamann atop Cliff Creek Ridge with the Bighorn Crags in the background.

behavior and population characteristics, patterns of fire and climate, and the introduction of endangered species. Terry was interested in all these aspects of the ranch, and he anticipated his time there. As a scientist, he had learned to appreciate the unique opportunities the ranch afforded. Greeted by the ranch managers, Terry felt comfortable and at ease, particularly when he saw the big gray mare he'd be riding up the mountain.

"She looks like a calm one," Terry thought to himself—not that he was an inexperienced rider. He'd grown up around horses and felt comfortable in most any situation—at least he thought he did until that weekend.

The history of the Frank Church Wilderness Area is rich. Sheepeater Indians are thought to be the first to reside there, attracted by the abundant natural resources such as bighorn sheep, mule deer, Chinook salmon, spring steelhead, cutthroat trout, and many species of riparian berries. The round depressions from their house pits can be seen

The sixty-five-acre Taylor Ranch is nestled between the Middle Fork of the Salmon River and Big and Monumental Creeks, thirty-six miles from the nearest road.

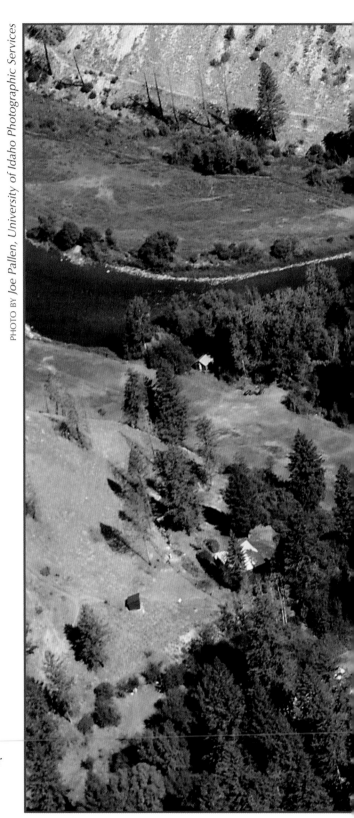

PHOTO BY Joe Pallen, University of Idaho Photographic Services

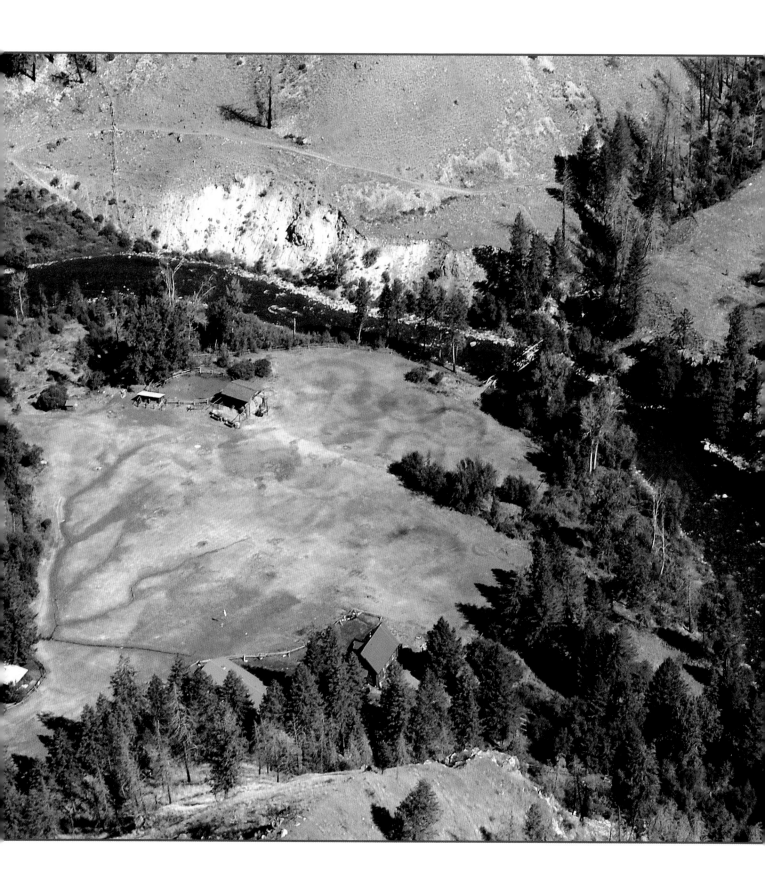

today. The Sheepeater Indian War of 1879 was the last Indian war fought in the Pacific Northwest. In July of that year, General O. Howard dispatched seventy-six men from Boise to investigate accusations that the Indians were stealing horses and causing trouble. The pursuit and ensuing battles through the mountainous terrain during the next several months were difficult for the Boise soldiers, who were unprepared for six-foot snow drifts and rough terrain. Finally, on October first, fifty-one Indian men, women, and children were captured and resettled on the Fort Hall Reservation. A few small bands remained in the area, having eluded the army, and continued to live their mountain life unmolested in its ancient pattern for another decade or two.

For many years, the Taylor Ranch site was known as the Lewis Place, owned by "Cougar Dave" Lewis, the quintessential Idaho frontiersman. He made a living off the land hunting, trapping, panning for gold, and growing a large garden and hay crop. He also guided hunters into the region.

In 1934, Jess Taylor purchased the ranch from Lewis with the dream of making it a premier gust ranch. Thirty years later, University of Idaho Professor Maurice Hornocker began conducting mountain lion research from Taylor Ranch, developing a friendship with the owner. That friendship ultimately led to the sale of the ranch to the University of Idaho in 1970, with visions of it becoming a wilderness field station. Today, University of Idaho students spend summers at the ranch conducting research.

After Terry's plane landed that morning in 1988, the group stored their gear in the visitor's cabin, then set out on a well-traveled path along the steep mountainside. The gray mare was obviously familiar with the route and paced sure-footed in spite of the rocky outcrops, narrow trail, and Terry's six-foot-nine frame. The team joked and talked science along the way, pointing out some of the interesting geological phenomena that they encountered. Traversing a narrow trail cut into a mountainside can be unnerving, particularly knowing that one slip over the edge could be fatal. Terry recalls feeling a little anxious whenever the trail became treacherous. "But it was always just so amazing to break out onto a plateau and look across the mountains," he said.

When Terry's mare suddenly stopped on the trail, he initially couldn't figure out what her problem was. In spite of his attempt to get her going, she refused to budge. Terry knew horses enough to trust her instincts. He knew something was wrong. He was searching the ground ahead of him to see what was holding the horse up when he spotted a rattlesnake camouflaged in the grass close to the path up ahead. The other horses ahead of him hadn't even seen it.

"The gray mare was totally calm with the snake," said Terry. "She was the only one who saw it. She calmly stopped and seemed to say, 'Is someone going to take care of this?'"

That was Terry's second inclination that he was riding a good horse. He had encountered many rattlesnakes in his time, but never on horseback. He was amazed at how calm the horse remained. He called ahead to the group. They dismounted and walked back to where the snake was hiding, taking that opportunity to discuss the different types of rattlesnakes that inhabited the area. Finally Terry walked over, pinned the snake with a stick, and picked it up. After showing it to the other travelers, he tossed it away from the trail and remounted his horse. He was anxious to get moving and eager to get to the mountaintop. By now he could hear distant thunder rumbling.

The group continued along the narrow path up the mountain toward their final destination: an overlook of a Bighorn Sheep habitat. But before long it was evident they were heading into a fierce storm. The thick, rolling thunderheads darkened the sky and soon the group realized they needed to take cover somewhere to avoid a downpour. By now, thunder boomed across the mountains, echoing from peak to peak, and every few minutes a bolt of lightning lit up the sky. In a few minutes, the group was smack in the middle of the raging electrical storm. They realized they needed to get back down the mountain and out of the weather. But once the rain began, the trail quickly became muddy and slippery. Terry began to feel a mounting panic. Still, the gray mare forged ahead, unaffected by any of the surrounding elements and her passenger's fear.

What happened next was a rare phenomenon few people have ever witnessed. Suddenly a huge spherical ball of blue light thundered and rolled down the mountainsides, lasting several seconds as the *boom! boom!* reverberated over and over. The sound was deafening, but the sight was extraordinary—unlike anything Terry had ever seen. He was now even more terrified. Never before had he seen such a thing. He stopped his horse and watched the scene before him with awe. He was tense and began to feel a rising panic. Most horses, when realizing their passenger is terrified, will also become terrified. But the gray mare didn't flinch.

"What the heck was that?" Terry yelled above the noise after the other riders had calmed their horses and themselves.

"Ball lightning," someone yelled out.

Ball lightning is not the same as lightning bolts, but is a spherical luminous object that appears in the sky during thunderstorms. Its existence is so rare that its reality has been controversial and even regarded as a fantasy or a hoax in the past. Due to inconsistencies in data, the exact nature of ball lightning is still unknown.

"I've never seen anything like it," said Terry. "But the most amazing thing was how the mare reacted. She was quite remarkable. I think of that trip often. The way she stood calmly during all that turmoil was really amazing. Had she spooked and run off in that steep rocky terrain, or fallen over the edge, it's hard to know what our fate would have been." In places along that trail, the fall to the bottom of the mountain seems neverending.

As the group maneuvered their way back down the mountain, they each knew they had encountered something special and terrifying on the mountain. It was an experience they would never forget.

When Terry flew out of Taylor Ranch a couple of days later, he took two things with him: the memory of ball lightning—an amazing phenomenon that few encounter—and thoughts of the big gray mare, who stayed totally calm in the presence of danger. Even now, more than twenty years later, he has few words to describe his experiences that August day. When he starts to think of it, he looks off into space for several seconds before speaking.

"It was all really quite remarkable," he'll say. "Really quite remarkable."

MOJO:
A LITTLE BIT OF MAGIC

—— Penny Kocher ——

"Opportunity had knocked, but now I was faced with a difficult choice. Was I willing to open that door, knowing full well it could be the end of my marriage?"

I was a typical horse-crazy woman. But, perhaps like many other women, I was married to someone who didn't understand my love of horses. Although I longed for a horse my entire life, at thirty-three years old and with two children of my own, I had still never owned one. I graduated from an equine college, worked for an Olympic show jumper, and ridden in competitive trail rides. In spite of my involvement with horses, I still held fast to my dream of owning my own.

Over the years I had begged for and borrowed every horse available. Everyone who knew me was aware of what horses meant to my life. Luckily, I had friends who wholeheartedly supported my horse hobby and let me pretend that their horses were my own. They allowed me free rein with all their horses. I rode their draft mare and even halter-broke the filly their old mare had. I brushed and rode and got to smell horses every week—and horse lovers know that's an important part of loving horses. But it wasn't enough. They even offered me free board if I ever did get the chance to make my dream come true. But still, it wasn't the same as if it were my own horse.

The only reason I didn't own a horse was because of my relationship with my husband. My husband and I had grown apart over the years and had fallen out of love several years before. But staying married was easier than the unknown of separation and divorce with two small children. I felt old and depressed most of the time, and my love of horses and the need to have them in my life had become a bone of contention between us over the years. He simply could not tolerate the fact that I loved horses.

Sunday mornings were the best part of my week. My husband would leave for golf, and my two small children and I would walk over to the local Standardbred harness racetrack. We did this every week to get my horse "fix," and of course we had our favorites that we would stop to pet. The big bay noses that peeked over those stall doors were like a balm to sooth my soul. The trainers and owners came to know us and got used to seeing us wander down the aisles, just looking or stopping to talk for a few minutes. The trainers would talk to my children and let them feed treats to some of the horses.

Sunday, July 9, 2006, is the day that forever changed my life. One of the trainers asked me if I wanted a horse.

"What? Are you serious?" I said.

"Today I'm giving them away," he replied.

It turns out he was looking to re-home a three-year-old mare that wasn't fast enough to race. He didn't want any money for her; he just wanted her to go to a good home. She was completely sound and had given him her all, but she just couldn't make the times required for the races. He said he could sell her to the Mennonites for a few hundred dollars, or he could give her to me, a family that he knew would love and care for her.

In this part of the country Mennonite horses are resources that are generally hard used and not to be fussed over. The mare's future would be uncertain. How could I allow that to happen when I had the opportunity to take this horse as my own?

Free horse and free board . . . if this wasn't fate I don't know what is! Opportunity had knocked, but now I was faced with a difficult choice. Was I willing to open that door, knowing full well it could be the end of my marriage?

For the sum of one whole dollar, to make it legal, I was suddenly the very proud owner of one beautiful Standardbred pacing mare. I call her Mojo, which means "a little bit of magic." Because that is exactly what she brought into my life.

I took Mojo to my friend's place the next day after picking her up straight off the racetrack. She loaded and came off the trailer like a pro; she was excited but not unmanageable. I didn't know a thing about her personality, but if this was any indication, I knew I had a good horse on my hands.

I started retraining her myself. Getting her used to the saddle was no problem, and she had already been bridled. But I remember the day I first put my leg over her and my weight on her back—I was scared silly that she would buck or bolt or something. Instead, she walked around like we'd been doing it forever. She was a definite keeper!

I felt really good about things and started to push her training a bit. That's where I got in over my head. She discovered rearing, like the black stallion with hooves reaching for the sky. So for a while, because of my fear, she became a pasture ornament. I still played and fussed with her, but I had lost my confidence and began to question if I should even own a young, athletic horse. But there was no way I was willing to give up on a dream that I had longed for so many years.

Then, three months after I got Mojo, my husband said our marriage was over.

I was ready for it; he had only said the words I was too much of a coward to say, and we parted as friendly as any divorcing couple could. I took our two small children and within two weeks bought a small brick house in a wonderful neighborhood. It was a new beginning for us. Mojo still stayed with my friends, but now we had all the time in the world to visit with her.

I was a rusty rider and she was a green mare—not a great combination. I didn't ride her myself much for a while, but she would very happily give my kids pony rides all day while I led her around. That would have been enough for me, just to see the smiles on my children's faces. My children would come into the barn, and she would lower her head and place it gently into their arms for a rub. She was most definitely worth her one dollar in those moments.

As a single parent, I had to watch my money closely. Finally having my own horse but not being able to really ride her gave me a focus and a goal. After all the bills were paid, I discovered I had enough money left over from my Christmas bonus to send Mojo to a trainer. I took her to a wonderful woman who runs a riding school and 4-H barn. She gives lessons to children and adults and trains horses using natural horsemanship methods. She honestly has the patience of Job. She understood my fears and knew what to do about Mojo's rearing issues. She did as much to train me as she did to train Mojo.

For six months I took lessons on her school horses while she trained Mojo. Finally, I was ready to ride my girl on my own. Those first few rides were scary. We ran the gambit of green horse tactics—bucking, biting, and balking. There were times I doubted my ability and my sanity. But we endured. Mojo taught me about patience and persistence. She has given me confidence in my horse skills. We built a strong bond, and with her I became a better, stronger person. She gave me a strong purpose throughout the difficult time of learning the art of independence and single parenting.

Since my divorce, I reconnected with my best friend in high school. He encourages me to spend time with my Mojo and even joins me at the barn sometimes for a ride. He accepts everything that makes me who I am, including my love of horses.

I really feel that Mojo was the catalyst to my new life. I saved her from an unknown situation, and she saved me from my unhappiness. Being part of her re-training has made me believe in my self-worth and my abilities. I believe in fate and good karma—Mojo is both. We are a team, and she will stay with me forever. My new life, in which with Mojo plays a very big part, makes me feel young and strong and alive again. I might tease Mojo that she isn't worth her dollar, but I wouldn't sell her for the entire world.

PENNY

— *Elaine Talley* —

"I struggled until I didn't have any more strength.

It was no use. I finally just sat down in the mud, exhausted.

I didn't know what to do."

Today is the first day I've been away from my house in almost five months. I have had agoraphobia most of my life. The longest I've been in the house without leaving is eight years. You see, I was severely abused as a child, and for many years I could not even speak and could barely move. I looked down at my feet most of the time. I felt frozen in time.

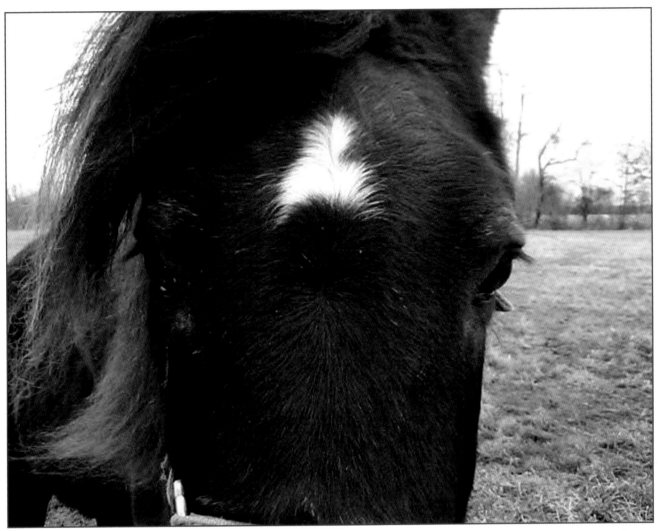

Elaine with her new friend, Buck. After Penny passed away, she befriended this neighbor horse.

It is through animals that I finally learned to communicate and through a little sorrel Quarter Horse named Penny that I learned to understand the love and faithfulness of a horse. Telling her story is a healing process for me.

I don't have human children, but I am a critter mom. I have rescued animals my whole life. I surround myself with wildlife and critters. They make me feel happy in this sad world I live in. I feel safe when I'm with them. They are my family.

I am also an artist—sandblast art, oil on canvas, as well as acrylic and watercolor. I also make Native American art such as beading, historically correct items, and other types of Native American art.

My husband and I moved to this old farmhouse to get away from the memories of the little town where I grew up. This home used to be in an old apple orchard. I still have the sign left here by the former owners that says APPLES FOR SALE. When we moved here, I had thirty-five cats and five dogs. I had a teepee up until recently, when the Ohio weather destroyed it. It took me many months of cursing and sewing by hand and machine to make it, but I was proud of it.

I go hiking every chance I get, when I'm not afraid to go outdoors. Whenever I encounter wildlife while hiking, they seem to know me and are not afraid, as they nonchalantly go about their day foraging and hunting for food. Some strange things have happened in my wildlife encounters. They just seem to know me and accept my presence while I'm in their world.

Right now, I'm down to just a few domestic critters. I feel lost and unprotected without them! Last year I lost my very protective pet steer named Moo Cow. He weighed over two thousand pounds. I also lost my very sweet dog named LooLoo. The very same week I also lost a kitty named Shelby Foot and a wild starling I had for twelve years, who even imitated the human voice! They are all gone now, and I miss them so. But more than any of them, I miss my sweet horse, Penny.

Penny was a red sorrel Quarter Horse who was very old when I got her. I had her about seven years before she died from old age. She had a scar across her nose from someone leaving the halter on her when she was growing up. I owned her long enough for me to understand that sixth sense horses have and the healing power that comes from it. We had some amazing experiences together.

One of my husband's friends was going to move, so his wife reluctantly let me have Penny because she knew I would take good care of her. When I got Penny, I wasn't familiar with horses at all, nor had I ever owned one. She was only about 14-hands high, with a very swayed back. The woman who gave her to me just handed me the

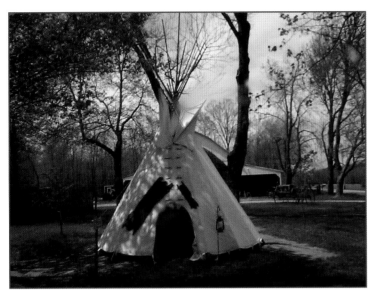

Elaine made this teepee to help herself heal.

lead rope with Penny attached to the other end, munching away on green grass in my front lawn. That was in 1990.

In Penny's last days, it was really cold, and I didn't have anything to keep her warm, so I wrapped myself around her and sang to her. My sweet Penny died on February 3, 1997. I was so lonely back then. I could hardly speak or understand folks when they spoke to me. Penny always leaned against me when I stood there and talked with her. She treated me like one of her foals, and I felt in a way like I was her child.

I grew to know Penny well, but I never got on her back. For some reason I just couldn't find it in my heart to put a bit in her mouth or treat her like a work animal. So I chose not to get on her or ride her. It didn't take long for Penny to figure me out. She was always there when I was in trouble. When I was out in the yard or when a stranger came by, she wanted to know who was here.

Some types of men seem to seek out vulnerability. One day a man came by the house. I wasn't speaking well at the time, and he realized this quickly in the few moments we spoke. He tried to get me into the barn, and I was too vulnerable to understand what he was trying to do. Penny tried to stomp him to death! I thought, "She's never done this before. What's wrong with my horse?"

That's just one of the many stories about how Penny looked out for me. But one incident in particular really amazes me whenever I think about it.

I was out in back of the barn early one morning trying to clear the muddy path that leads to the barn for Penny. I had my knee-high rubber boots on as I cleared away the muck. I was home alone, and there were no houses close by at that time. It was very quiet as I worked, although I did hear the sweet sound of wild birds singing, and I glanced up to watch them as I dug. Penny was in the pasture not too far away, eyeing me nonchalantly as she always did, making sure I was okay.

I guess I didn't realize how muddy it really was, because suddenly I sank knee-high in the muck and couldn't move. Like a suction cup, the mud grabbed on to my legs and wouldn't let me go. I struggled to get out, but the boots were too tight to slide off my feet. I started to panic because I knew that it would be many hours before my husband got home—and it was getting chilly outside. I struggled until I didn't have any more strength. It was no use. I finally just sat down in the mud, exhausted. I had no idea what to do.

Suddenly Penny walked over to me and dropped her head down. My first thought was that she was sick. I thought, *Oh Penny, don't be sick now—please!* There was no way I could help her if she was sick. Penny stood quietly with her head on my chest for several minutes. I stroked her head and ears and talked to her, thinking she was ill. While having her there was comforting, I was also really worried about her.

Then I thought, 'I might as well take advantage of her standing here.' So I reached up and wrapped my arms around her head and pulled. As soon as I had a good hold, Penny slowly raised her head. She didn't stop pulling until I was completely free of the mud. It wasn't until she pulled me upward that I was finally able to pull my feet out of the boots. Wide eyed and full of disbelief and amazement at what was happening, I tucked my legs up, and she carried me out and away from the mud and began to

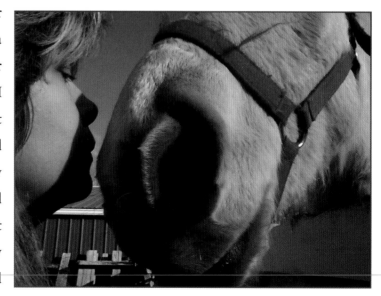

Elaine and a neighbor horse, Dillon.

shake. I dropped to the ground like a rock. Penny nuzzled me for a second, then she walked off as if nothing had happened.

I realized then that Penny wasn't sick at all; she just knew I had been in trouble, and she intended all along to help me. I wish I had a video of this whole thing. It is so amazing to me that a horse would do that for me.

When Penny started to fail, Moo Cow stood with her to the end. It was the hardest thing in the world to let her go, but she was over forty years old. I called the vet out, and he gave her a shot to perk her up, but she only lasted a week after that. I'll say it again—it was the hardest thing in the world to let her go. But I am so grateful for what she taught me and the love that she showed me.

All I've ever wanted to do in life was to give the animals the dignity and respect they deserve. Too many people neglect and abuse them.

Since Penny's death, I've met and befriended a few horses not my own. I've spent many hours in the pasture with an old soul of a horse in need, through the wind and rain and snowstorms and ice, shielding his head from the elements. This wonderful old stallion had no shelter or windbreak at all—just an empty pasture with no tree to shelter him. This horse I speak of even knew my sweet Penny. They had a few little rendezvous in the night without my permission. They really liked each other and would whinny across the way at each other. I can still hear the echo of their friendly calls to each other on those warm summer days.

All my critters are getting old and passing on, but I still have a coon hound named Emmaline, a mini donkey named Donkey Bill, a little white goat named Itchy, and six kitty cats. But in spite of their protection and companionship, I still miss my little sorrel Quarter Horse named Penny.

LITTLE BUDDY

—— Ivy Christian ——

"Time literally stopped for me at

that terrifying moment."

My niece, Michelle, often came over from her home on the Washington coast to spend time with family in Idaho. I'm her aunt, but also kind of her second mother. I got her hooked on horses, which was really good for her because she was dealing with some tough issues in life. She started out riding my Quarter Horse, Skippy, whom she adored.

When Michelle was seventeen years old, she drove over one weekend to see us and go riding. This was after I'd bought a cutting horse, and we spent a lot of time practicing in the cutting pen with a mechanical cow. I knew that my cutting horse, Little Buddy, was a hot little cookie but also felt that he was fairly safe. After we worked the cutting horses this particular weekend, Michelle asked to ride Buddy down to the barn—which was only about hundred feet away at the most. I thought she would be fine.

PHOTO BY *Cheryl Dudley*

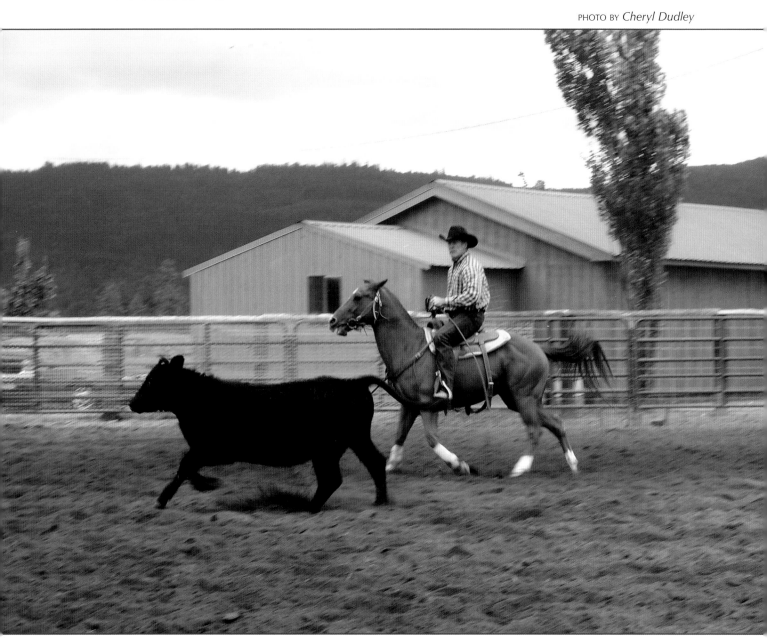

Little Buddy cutting at a regional show in Idaho

My first mistake was not shortening the stirrups for her. She had such a short distance to go, I didn't want to bother, and I assumed the two would be fine. Mistake number two: I thought that Michelle was far enough along to be able to ride him.

When Michelle and Buddy started down a small incline toward the barn, the stirrups began bumping Buddy's sides. Buddy thought she was asking him to go—so he took off. He was just doing what he'd been taught to do. Michelle didn't have her reins short, so I yelled, "Michelle, shorten your reins, shorten your reins!"

Then she panicked. Now not only were the stirrups banging him, but she also gripped him with her feet. To Buddy, that meant, "Go!" They went down around the barn, and Michelle was trying to get him stopped, pulling on the reins and yelling. Her yelling only added to the excitement level. They disappeared down over the hill, and I heard Buddy's hooves loping away on the packed driveway. A terrifying vision began to form in my mind.

Our house sat about a quarter mile off a busy, windy, and very hilly highway. As the horror of what could happen struck me, my mind raced. I screamed to my partner, "Go after her!" So he took off at a trot after her. By then it was too late.

It was a quiet summer Sunday evening and, thank God, there were no chip trucks on the highway, because the next thing I heard was horseshoes clopping on pavement.

Oh no—they had reached the highway!

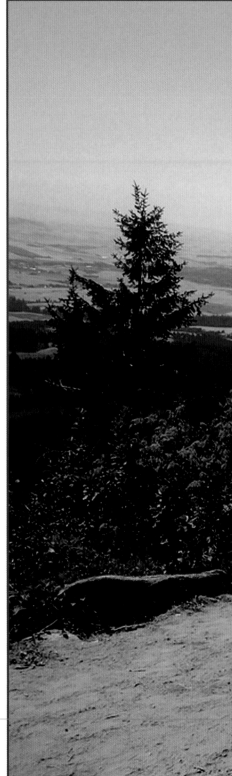

PHOTO BY Cheryl Dudley

Little Buddy and his new owner, Don Dudley ➢

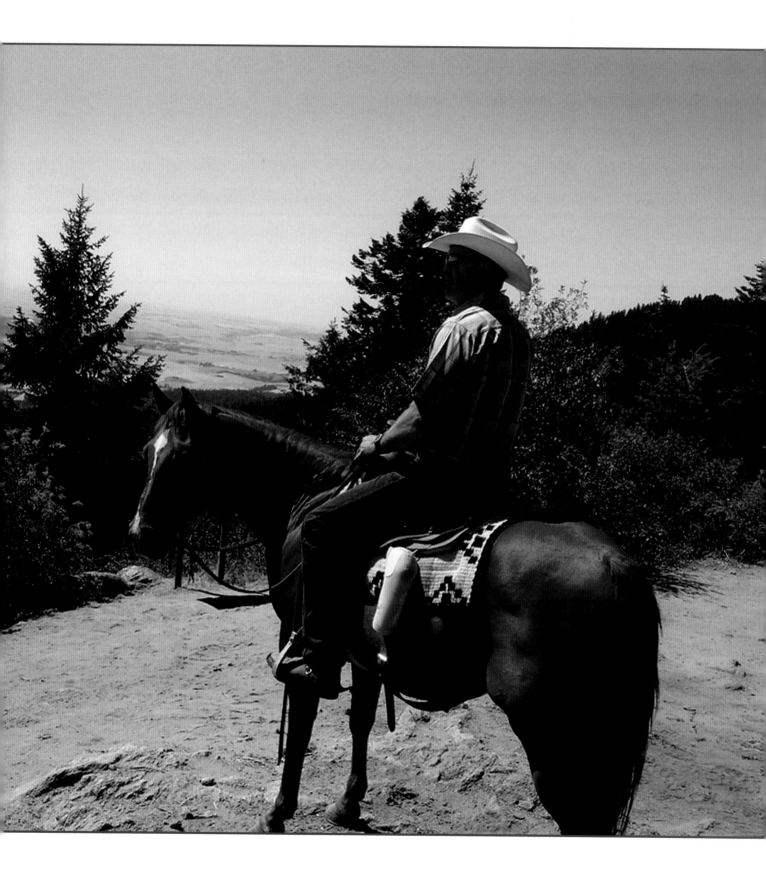

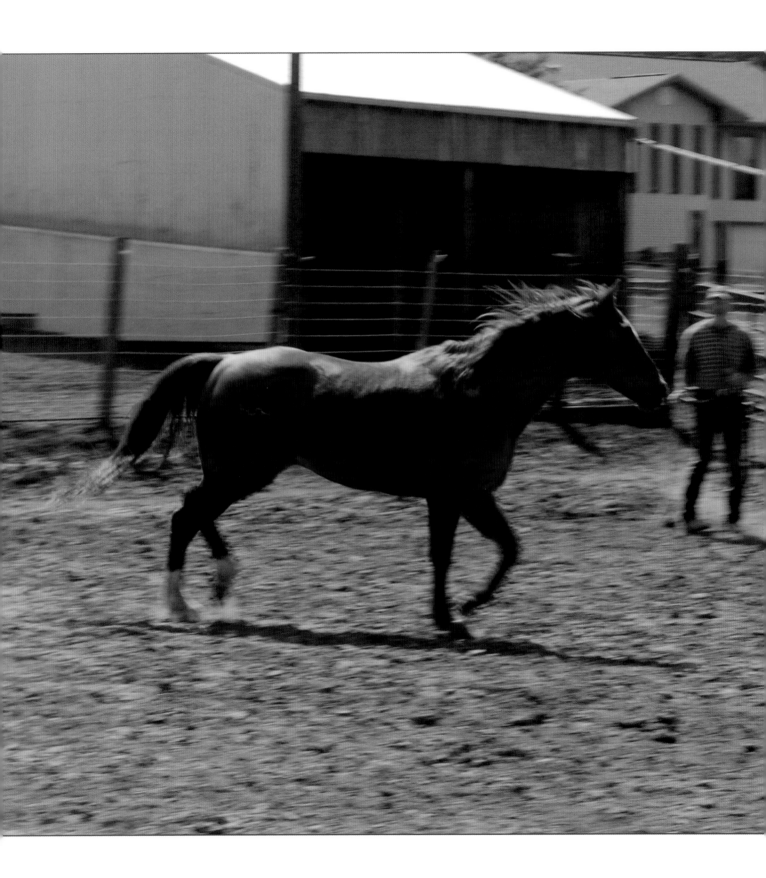

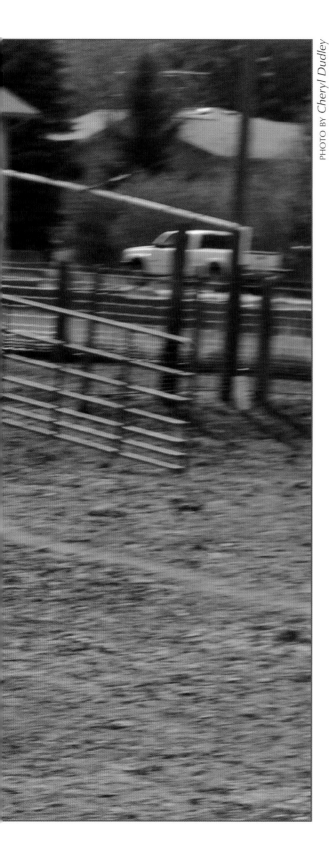

PHOTO BY *Cheryl Dudley*

Time literally stopped for me at that terrifying moment. I jumped in my pickup, drove out to the highway, and looked up the hill. I couldn't see anything. I pulled out onto the highway and crested the south hill and looked down the other side. Buddy and Michelle were already at the bottom of the hill—about a half mile away.

Two days earlier, Buddy had been freshly shod. Steel horseshoes on asphalt are not a good combination. To Buddy, it was like trying to stop while going full speed downhill on an ice skating rink. At the speed he was running, it was all he could do to stay upright. Michelle was crouched down, hanging tightly to the saddle horn, with her legs and feet clamped tightly around Buddy's belly. He interpreted that as her desire for him to keep going. Several times he did try to slow down and stop, but when he did, his feet would slide. His back pasterns gave way and slid along the asphalt several time, searing off his flesh to the bone. But thankfully he was always able to right himself. He was taking good care of his terrified rider.

Partway down the hill, a car approached from behind, and the driver called out to Michelle. "Do you need help?"

◄ Playing hard to get

Michelle nodded her head yes. So the driver drove up beside Buddy and slowly eased him over toward the guardrail. When he got to the bottom of the hill on more solid footing, Buddy was finally able to come to a stop. His hooves were so hot they were literally smoking. And Michelle was hyperventilating. But the two seemed to be okay.

By the time I got to the bottom of the hill, Buddy was sweating, but calm. As a matter of fact, he seemed fairly unaffected by the whole incident. After all, he was only doing what he was asked to do. It's a miracle he never fell down. If he had—well, we are not sure if either he or Michelle would have survived a long skid along the asphalt coupled with possible passing vehicles. At the very least they would have been severely injured.

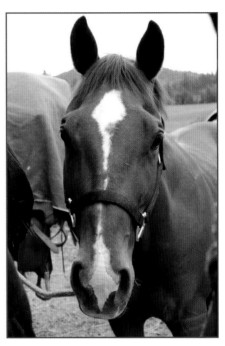

Little Buddy

Buddy spent the next eight months in his stall. Each day I took the bandages off his back legs and picked the pieces of asphalt out of his wounds. The day after the incident, I called the farrier out to remove the shoes he'd put on two days before. They were worn down to about an eighth of an inch and had melted into his hoof walls.

For the next three months, whenever I drove over that hill I could see Buddy's skid marks going down the side of the highway, and I said a little prayer of thanks. Because of his courage, athleticism, and heart, Little Buddy saved not only his own life, but my niece's life as well.

About Ivy

Ivy Christian grew up in Washington State and has spent her entire life around horses. She currently works for Pullman Transit and competes in local and regional cutting horse shows.

FLICKA, DINA, AND A MULE NAMED PINKY

— *Don Dudley* —

Don recalled something his dad had told him:

"Whenever you're in trouble, give your horse his head, keep him

between your legs, and he'll take care of you."

The Dudley children—Dennis, Bud, Don, Duke, and Diane—grew up in the Frank Church Wilderness Area on the main Salmon River in Idaho. Homeschooled by their mother, Jennie, the children had more freedom than most, along with acres of wide-open spaces to roam and try out their wings. They grew up learning how to be coordinated and savvy in the wilderness, whether it was fishing the clear whitewater creeks that flowed into the Salmon or riding with a pack string into the mountains with their father, Harold.

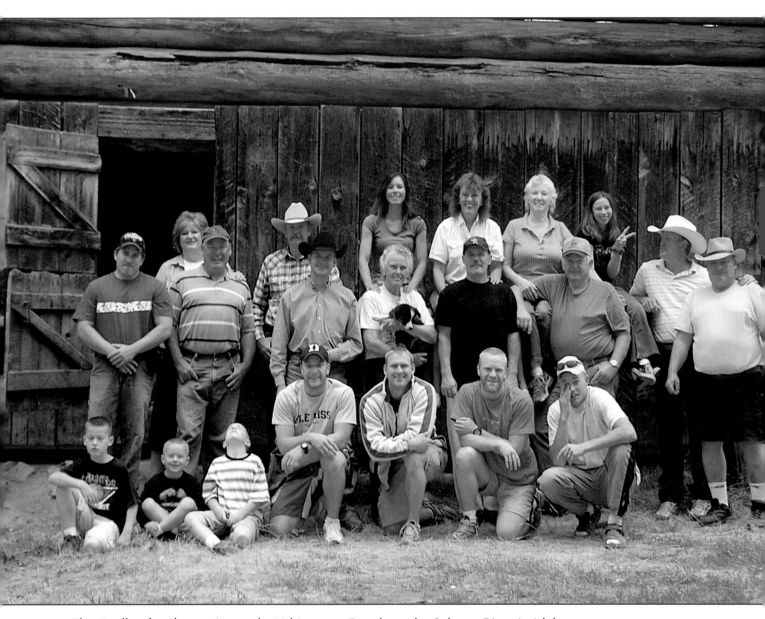

The Dudley family reunion at the Whitewater Ranch on the Salmon River in Idaho

The family owned a ranch on the river that they named the Whitewater Ranch, where they operated an outfitting business for hunters who traveled there from all over the United States. The hunting and packing experiences were one of a kind, set apart by the rushing whitewater of the Salmon River, the steep narrow trails that led into no-man's-land, and the home-cooked meals of Jennie Dudley. Hunting trips at the Whitewater Ranch were carefully planned and executed to provide hunters a safe, productive, and fulfilling experience. Those years were the best for the Dudley family.

The family owned a string of solid horses and pack mules that were bombproof. The five children would get up early in the morning to feed and tend to the animals before sitting down to school lessons for a few hours each weekday. The rest of their time was spent exploring or helping out their parents with the multiple chores necessary to keep up the ranch, whether it be milking the cows, feeding the pigs, riding into the mountains to herd horses, or fishing the snow-fed creeks that rushed down the mountains into the Salmon River.

Diane, the only girl in the family, was the youngest of the five children. Next up was Duke, then Don, Bud, and Dennis, the eldest. The Dudley children learned how to plan for week-long pack trips into the wilderness, how to negotiate the narrow rocky trails that cut into the mountainside, and to trust their horse's instincts and surefootedness. These skills became essential and perhaps life-saving at times.

In the fall of 1962, when Don was eleven years old and Duke was ten, the family led a hunting group into the Chamberlain Basin area, where they stayed at base camp for a week and ventured out to hunt during the day. Base camp—consisting of several large wall tents—had been established for the season, and it provided shelter, supplies and cooking utensils for the seven- to ten-day hunting expeditions.

At the end of each hunting trip, the group rode twenty-three miles back down to the ranch to pick up another hunting group that would be waiting. On this particular trip in 1962, Don and Duke begged their father to let them stay at base camp alone for the weekend, from Friday to Monday, while the rest of the group rode back to the ranch. Their father agreed, knowing that the boys were experienced and would know how to care for themselves. The hunters rode out that morning with the pack string to return to the ranch, leaving the two boys behind with two dogs, Don's horse Flicka and Duke's little white mule named Pinky.

At first the boys were excited to be left alone at camp. They explored and bantered back and forth with each other. But a few hours after the hunters left, for some reason, the two became homesick.

< 97 >

"The dogs kept whining because they wanted to go home," said Don. "We wanted to keep them there, but finally we gave in to their whining. We decided we should go home." So with Don out front on Flicka and Duke following on Pinky, the boys began the long, twenty-three-mile, eight-hour trip home, knowing that the day would grow dark before they arrived.

About an hour down the trail, Don and Duke came upon one of the ranch horses, named Dina, along the trail. Dina did not get along well with the other horses, so the boys assumed their father had let her go somewhere along the way, knowing she would eventually find her own way home. They decided to catch her and lead her home. Unaware, they tied their mounts near a bee nest while they took out after Dina. In a few moments, Flicka and Pinky began to buck and carry on. By then, Don and Duke had caught Dina, and they ran over and rescued the horse and mule.

They mounted and continued their ride home, Don ponying Dina behind Flicka, and Duke following on Pinky.

Before long, the boys understood why their father had let Dina go. She hated Pinky walking behind her and started to kick at her. Finally, one of her kicks caught Duke square on his shin.

"He didn't cry at first, even though he said it hurt," said Don.

The two stopped for a moment while Duke rubbed his shin. Soon he said he was fine. Feeling the urgency of time, they continued down the trail.

About an hour later, Duke said he felt something warm in his boot and told Don his leg hurt. Don dismounted and tied the horses, then walked back to check it out. When they pulled up Duke's pant leg, they saw that the cut was severe and bleeding profusely into Duke's boot—and they couldn't get the boot off.

Duke started to cry. Don took the scarf from around his neck and tied it around Duke's leg to stop the bleeding. They continued down the trail. By now it was dark.

A few miles up ahead, an elderly woman named Francis Zaunmiller, who was a writer, lived in a tiny cabin. Her husband had passed away, and Francis lived alone. The boys knew her well, so they decided to stop in and ask for her help with Duke's injury. She answered the door and rushed the boys inside. She looked at Duke's leg with concern. "We'll need to soak this in water to get the boot off," she said. After settling Duke, she called the boys' parents on her old three-party crank phone to tell them what had happened.

The Dudleys decided that Don should ride on home leading Dina, but that Duke should stay with Francis for the night. Dina was too cranky to pen up with the other

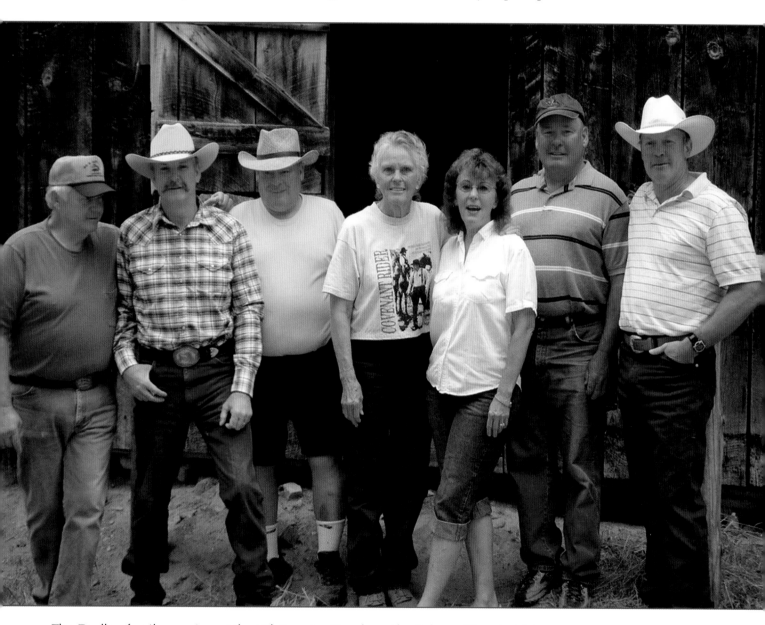

The Dudley family reunion at the Whitewater Ranch on the Salmon River in Idaho
From left: Jennie's brother, Herb Vloedman, Duke, Dennis, Jennie, Diane, Bud, and Don

horses, and she needed to be brought home. All these years later, Don justifies that as the reason he was told to ride home. The Zaunmiller cabin was only four miles from the Whitewater Ranch—but four of the most treacherous miles.

As the realization of his task sunk in, Don had several misgivings, even though he'd ridden the narrow trail along the river numerous times.

"Francis reminded me of the white-haired lady in the Hansel and Gretel story," said Don. "And even though Duke annoyed me at times, I wasn't sure I wanted to leave him alone with her, to an unknown fate."

But in spite of his fears, Don knew he needed to start home right away. He looked at his brother as he walked out the door.

"We'll be back to get you in the morning," he said, gathering up his jacket. As he mounted his horse, he recalled something his dad had told him: "Whenever you're in trouble, give your horse his head, keep him between your legs, and he'll take care of you."

Darkness had completely engulfed the deep canyon as Don, Flicka, and Dina negotiated the one-lane suspension bridge that crossed the Salmon River. Once on the other side, the trail was cut into steep rock cliffs that dropped straight into the rushing water. Don was getting sleepy as night fell, particularly after the trauma of his brother's injury. But he wasn't afraid. As he rocked back and forth with the rhythm of Flicka's steps, he began to close his eyes occasionally just for a short rest.

Before long, he could see nothing, but he knew from experience that horses could see well in the dark.

"I tried to watch the trail," said Don. "Once, I thought the trail went to the right, so I was kind of leaning that way, when Flicka suddenly went left. I had been wrong. From that moment on, I looked down, closed my eyes, held onto the saddle horn, and just rocked with the rhythm of the horse. I thought about all the fun things I liked to do, like hunt and fish. I wouldn't have wanted to walk home because I couldn't have seen the trail. Every time I'd fall asleep and start to slide off the saddle, Flicka would kind of jerk and wake me up," said Don.

When Don finally rode into the ranch on Flicka late that night, he didn't think much about how the horse had safely delivered him home. He was just glad to be there. It wasn't until many years later that he realized the gravity of what had happened that night.

And of course Duke was fine the next day when they rode back down the river to Mrs. Zaunmiller's cabin to retrieve him for the trek back up to base camp.

Two years later the Dudley family moved out of the wilderness to start a logging business. Looking back on their experiences at the Whitewater Ranch, the Dudley children feel blessed that they had such amazing experiences that equipped them to face life's many hardships.

The summer of 2007, for the first time since moving away from the ranch, the family got together at the Whitewater Ranch for a family reunion. Harold had long since passed away, but Jennie made arrangements to get there from her home in Utah. All five of the children were there, including their children and grandchildren.

As the family crossed the narrow bridge that spanned the river and hiked up the trail that led to Francis Zaunmiller's cabin—now a famous historical site—Duke and Don recalled the night that Duke now calls "The Night of Abandonment" and got a good laugh.

When they reached the cabin, they recollected their memories of that night, and Don thought fondly of Flicka and the night she carried him home safely through the dark.

About Don

Don Dudley has been a practicing farrier for more than thirty years. He also coached basketball, football, and track for many years. He has a degree in education from the University of Idaho and has been involved in cutting for four years. In 2004, he purchased Ivy Christian's horse Little Buddy.

PANDA, THE SEEING EYE HORSE

— Ann Edie —

"When I pick up the harness, I get the feeling from her that I'm ready for anything. Let's go have fun."

Ann Edie was born with Leber's congenital amaurosis, a degenerative eye condition that over time results in severe vision loss. Although legally blind since birth, Ann was taught to read large print with the aid of heavy reading glasses. She depended mostly on her listening skills to learn throughout elementary school, high school, and while she earned her bachelor's degree and first master's degree. In the 1980s she taught herself Braille, and she later went on to earn a second master's degree.

While in graduate school in New Jersey, Ann met her husband Dennis. After graduation the two married and moved to Japan for three years, where Ann taught English as a second language and studied the Japanese language and Dennis worked as a chemist.

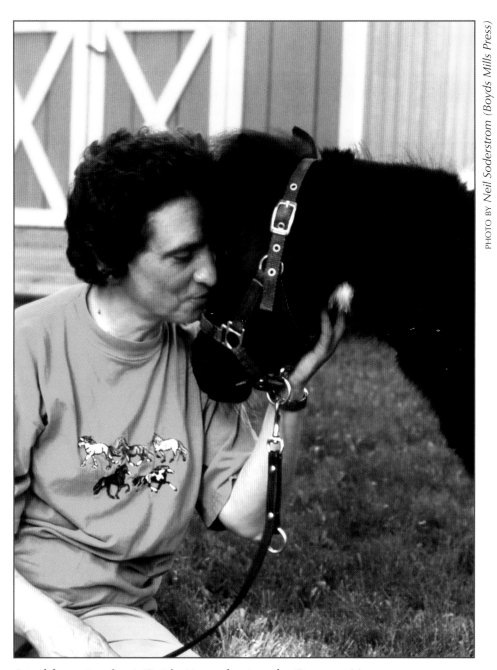

PHOTO BY *Neil Soderstrom (Boyds Mills Press)*

Reprinted from *Panda: A Guide Horse for Ann*, by Rosanna Hansen

From Japan, the couple moved to Taiwan, where their first son, Eric, was born. After having the baby, they decided to move back to the United States to be near family. Ann taught the Chinese language in Virginia and there gave birth to their second son, Wayne. In 1985, the family moved to New York, where their daughter, CarolAnn, was born. Ann stayed home with the children for a few years, but also taught English as a second language to recent immigrants.

In 1991, Anne's vision had become impaired enough that she decided to get a seeing eye dog. Bailey, a lovable chocolate Labrador, entered their lives. He was Ann's companion and a part of the family for nine years. During that time, Ann decided to become certified to teach the visually impaired, and she earned her second master's degree at Boston College.

In October 2000, Bailey died, leaving Ann heartbroken and in search of a new guide dog. Over the next two years, she tried out two different German Shepherd guide dogs, but neither dog worked out. They dragged her across lawns as they chased cats and squirrels and even pulled her into the street as they chased dogs in passing cars.

"It was a really frustrating time for me," said Ann. "Losing Bailey was an emotionally taxing experience. And establishing a new relationship with a guide animal takes a lot of emotional energy."

During this time, Ann had become close friends with Alexandra Kurland, author of books about the clicker training method for training horses, and she took horseback riding lessons from her. Alexandra saw what Ann was going through and felt bad about seeing her good friend so emotionally distraught.

Working together with a guide animal requires a partnership and a relationship of trust—something that takes from six months to a year to develop. The two need to learn to communicate in a way that works for both, and a good fit may not come naturally or easily. When Ann was unable to form a long-term partnership with the two German Shepherd dogs she had tried out, she decided to turn to a different animal for help.

She began reading about the Guide Horse Foundation, which was founded in 1999 as an experimental program to explore the abilities of miniature horses as guide animals. Being a horse lover, a new idea hatched in Ann's mind. What about training a miniature horse as her guide? She was no stranger to the horse-human bond, and the possibility of using a miniature horse to guide her, as opposed to a dog, intrigued her. Not only that, miniature horses are generally docile, strong, and not easily distracted.

The idea sounded more and more exciting to Ann.

So she approached Alexandra about the possibility of training a miniature horse guide for her using the clicker training method—a positive method that rewards desirable behavior in the animal, as opposed to punishing incorrect behavior. It didn't take long for Alexandra to agree.

Ann knew from her own experience that horses could be trained to do many of the things that guide dogs do for blind people. Her Arabian riding horse, Magnat, had already learned to stop at the barn doorway, stall doorway, and other places where Ann wanted to get oriented before going forward while she and Magnat were walking together around the farm where the horse lived. Magnat also knew that he needed to stop at places where they had to step up or over a tree root or threshold and he knows to lead Ann straight to the gate when she was taking him back to his paddock at night. When Ann was riding Magnat in the arena, she depended upon him to avoid obstacles like jumps and to navigate among other horses. And one of Magnat's favorite things to do was to fetch things that had been dropped in the arena, like a whip, a glove, or a hat, and bring them to Ann.

Other blind people have been known to ride alone on trails, completely relying on their horses to guide them. Given all this, it's not so unlikely that the miniature horse would be a perfect guide animal candidate.

Miniature horses are not ponies. Proportionately, they are like a regular-size horse—only much smaller. To be registered as a miniature horse, they cannot be taller than thirty-four inches at the withers. But miniature horses used as guides must

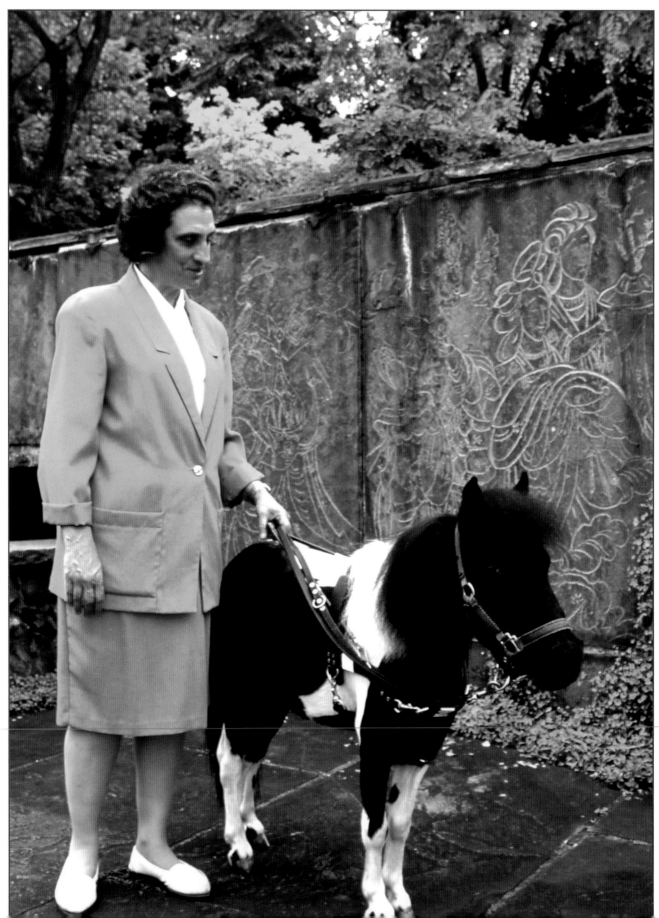

be even smaller—less than thirty inches tall—to conveniently fit into cars, public transportation, and places like restaurants, offices, and stores.

Small size is not the only qualification for miniature horses to become successful guide horses. They must also have a calm, confident, and friendly temperament. While small, they must also have good bone structure and excellent health, in order to have long and successful careers as guides.

One of the biggest advantages of miniature horses over dogs as guides is that they live much longer than dogs. They generally live between thirty and forty years. The prospect of building a partnership with a guide animal that could potentially last for decades instead of just a few years was very appealing to Ann.

After thoroughly researching the idea of using a miniature horse as a guide, Ann acquired a tiny, eight-month-old, black-and-white mini named Panda from a miniature horse farm in Florida. Alexandra began training her, and in 2003 Panda went to work for Ann full time, when she was just two and a half years old. Since then, the two have developed a strong bond and an outstanding working partnership.

Panda stands just twenty-nine inches tall and weighs only 120 pounds—no bigger than some large dogs. While Ann is capable of traveling using a white cane, she's grateful for the freedom and ease that Panda affords her in traveling independently. As a matter of fact, she says that Panda is the best guide she's ever had.

"Her guide work is really extraordinary," said Ann. "She's superb at obstacle avoidance and 100 percent accurate on curbs." One of the best benefits, however, is that after owning Panda for several years, their bond and communication continue to grow. If Panda were a dog, Ann would already be forced to think about a replacement animal because of her age. But instead, she can look forward to many more years of close partnership with Panda.

Miniature horses are mild-mannered and naturally cautious. They also have exceptional vision, with eyes set far apart, allowing a nearly 360-degree visibility range. Plus, they're herd animals, so they instinctively synchronize their movements

◄ Reprinted from *Panda: A Guide Horse for Ann*, by Rosanna Hansen

with others. A guide is trained to stop at changes in elevation, such as curbs and steps, to stay close to the left edge of roads without sidewalks, and to return to the edge after navigating around obstacles. They also find and indicate landmarks like doors, traffic signal buttons, and elevator buttons. They maneuver straight across a street to the opposite curb and will refuse to go forward into a street if there is any hazard in the way. If the handler tells the guide to go forward and there is a hazard, such as a car turning into the crosswalk, either the guide won't go forward or it will find a safe way around.

Panda is trained to do all these tasks and more. Plus she's house-trained.

"Panda is calm but aware of her environment," says Alexandra. "She's reliable and steady. She needs to eat and relieve herself more often than a dog, but when you think about having to train five to seven dogs in a lifetime as opposed to one or two horses, it's certainly worth it."

Ann really appreciates Panda's memory. "If I stop to show her a crosswalk signal button on Monday, Panda will take me directly to it on Tuesday," she reports. "I've found that horse intelligence lends itself well to guide work," she said.

"And Panda is a happy horse and loves her work," said Ann. "Part of that is the way she was trained, and part is because she is naturally curious and enjoys being with me out in the big world. She knows what she's supposed to do. When I pick up the harness, I get the feeling from her that, 'I'm ready for anything. Let's go have fun.'"

PATRICK

— Elizabeth Welch —

"During my depression, something strange kept happening. I kept having dreams about riding horses."

wo years ago I was entering the most important time in my life: I was planning my wedding. My brother had just returned home safely from a military tour in Iraq, and I was so grateful that he was home. We were finally all happily together again: my mother, father, sister, and brother. I was married on Valentine's Day 2007. It was one of the happiest days of my life.

But that happiness was short-lived.

On March 22, I was awakened early in the morning by a phone call. I was told that I needed to hurry to the hospital emergency room. My father had flatlined. When

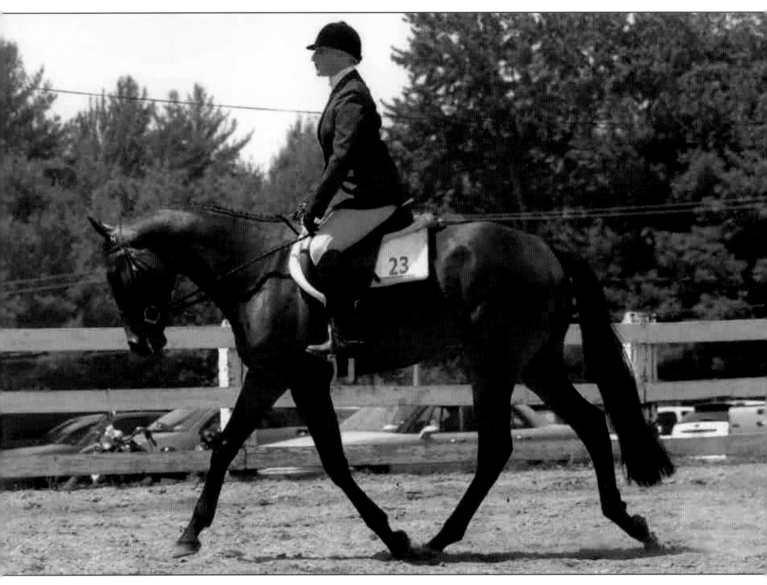

Elizabeth riding Patrick

I arrived, I watched in horror as the doctors administered CPR. Although he revived, his prognosis was grim.

For four days my family kept a constant vigil next to his bedside in the Intensive Care Unit as the doctors ran test after test. I watched as he breathed through a tube and experienced grand mal seizures. I held his hand and prayed for a miracle. But the miracle never happened. He had gone too long without oxygen and would never wake up.

My family made the decision to take my father off life support due to the extent of brain damage caused by lack of oxygen during his congestive heart failure. My brother, sister, and mother all watched our loved one slowly die before us. Our hearts were broken as we watched him struggle for life. I will never forget how I felt watching the once-strongest man in the world lay limp. It was March 26, 2007. I was devastated and heartbroken.

Eleven days later I was in the hospital losing my unborn child. The stress of losing my beloved father was just too much to bear. After I lost my baby, I found myself spiraling into a deep and lonely depression, missing my father and the way my family used to be: happy and safe and together.

During my depression, something strange kept happening. I kept having dreams about riding horses. In my dreams, my father was there watching me. It was very nice to see him again, even if it was just a dream. My recurring dream haunted me during the day, and I couldn't help but wonder if it was some sort of message.

I had ridden horses and taken lessons since I was seven years old and have loved horses as far back as I can remember. I'd always worked for my lessons at the riding facility near us, and in the summers I would be allowed a free lease on a green horse. It made me an experienced rider. I would have done anything just to be around horses back then. But when I headed off to college, bills and classes took precedence over horseback riding, and my love of horses took a temporary backseat to other things in life.

But now here I was, suddenly being drawn back to horses.

My vivid horse dreams continued, and I just couldn't get them off my mind. So I finally gave in. I bought a newspaper and saw an ad for a cheap lease. That was all I needed to get back in the saddle. It soothed my soul to be around a horse and start riding again. Yet I knew that I had to have more.

Leasing a horse held me over for a couple of months before I knew that I had to buy my own. I began my search with limited funds. One day I was at the local tack shop telling the owner I wanted to buy a Thoroughbred, but I didn't have over a thousand to spend. She got right on the phone for me.

The next thing I knew, my husband and I were driving out to ranches to look at horses. Although we'd looked at a few before this day, none fit my vivid dream. But today, luck would be on my side. I met the woman who was selling the horse. It turned out that I knew her from the riding facility where I had taken lessons for twelve years as a girl. I recalled how nice she was to the children and horses, and I felt that this meeting was promising.

The first horse she brought out was beautiful, but just too expensive. I explained to her my financial situation.

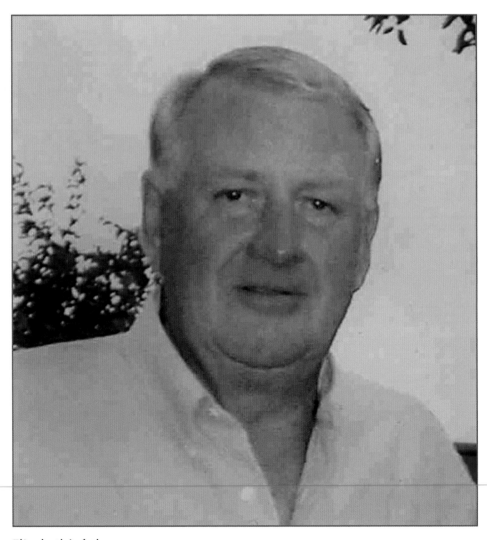

Elizabeth's father

"Okay, how about I show you Patrick?" she said. "He's in the far pasture because the other geldings were kind of beating him up, so he's alone. I haven't ridden him yet. He just came off the track a month ago."

When Patrick walked into the barn, it was truly love at first sight. I felt a warm tingly feeling ripple through my body. I touched his velvet muzzle and stared into his big, gentle brown eyes. I whispered to my husband, "He's the one."

"I can tell," he replied.

I rode him in an open field for a total of fifteen minutes. His gaits were smooth and floaty, and I felt that exhilaration I hadn't felt in years. We took him home, and on his back I began healing from the pain of loss. Patrick and I have been together ever since.

The dreams of my father watching me ride horses have stopped. It's almost as if he were guiding me in my dreams, telling me what I needed for the healing process. I know it is what he would have wanted for me.

I now have peace with my father's death because of Patrick. Whenever I ride, I know he's watching me.

A MEMOIR TO CLANCY

— *Cassey Cattell* —

"It's my firm belief that perfection is not what forms your love for something or someone. No. It's imperfections that make you love unconditionally, in an unexplainable manner."

My muse is running wild, and I'm missing you right now, Clancy. I imagine you moving smooth at a steady pace. I look at your ears and smile—thinking back to when this all began.

I was born with a mild condition of spastic dysplasia cerebral palsy, which is characterized by bent-knee walking due to tight leg muscles and weak trunk muscles. As a result, my parents were advised to sign me up for horseback riding as a form of therapy. I started riding as a small child at Fieldstone Farm Therapeutic Riding

Center in Chagrin Falls, Ohio, on a gorgeous little mare named Cricket, and I have ridden on and off since then. The thing I remember most about those early riding lessons years ago was being told to point our toes to the sky and look between our horse's ears. My young mind always took pleasure in that, for some reason. Whenever I was directly peering through Cricket's ears, I'd imagine I was heading toward some sort of target. Perhaps I was subconsciously driving myself toward a goal—I'm not sure. I still frequently dream of those lessons today.

I distinctly remember trotting together. Back then, the Western riding discipline was a choice here at Fieldstone, so I rode in a Western saddle. We got to cheat and hold on to the saddle horn when we were trotting, and it makes me laugh, thinking back on it. I loved to trot with Cricket. Something else that comes to mind was there was no scary lift! There was a huge ramp, and I'd walk up on it with my walker and hop on Cricket's back.

At any rate, I'm told that I grew "bored" with riding after about three years, though I'm not entirely sure I believe that. For the next five years I attended weekly physical therapy, and I clearly remember a constant longing to return to the saddle and continuous begging to do so. I'm not the most patient person in the world, but I'm sure everyone knows that, as the saying goes, good things come to those who wait.

For my eleventh birthday, my Gram, Kathy Cattell, gave me a card explaining that I would begin riding at Fieldstone again, paid for by her. It took a year to finally find a placement in the program that would fit my time schedule, but the summer before I turned twelve, I began riding at Fieldstone again. I started with instructor Tonya Zimmer and horse Banjo and then several months later was switched to a more convenient time slot with instructor Mary Hipp and horse Tonka—my first "baby."

I rode Tonka for about a year, and I loved him—he was one of those horses that didn't tolerate you unless he liked you, and from our first ride, he realized he wasn't going to intimidate me. For an old boy, he had the energy of a five-year-old. After Tonka came my big, sexy baby, Clancy. There isn't a thing I remember disliking about him, except perhaps his size. It was quite a stretch on my legs going from a Quarter Horse to a Thoroughbred-draft cross. By then I was working with instructor Bill Lavin.

Thus began the long and special partnership between Clance and I.

After about a year and a half with Bill, it was decided that I should move up to a more advanced level of riding, so I moved to Arlene Taylor's class. I tell Arlene all the time that she's a slave driver but that I love her for it. Between the three of us, I really did gain strength and improve so much as a rider.

Your sensitivities, Clancy, made me a better rider all around, with Arlene's help. At fifteen years old I was much more bold and opinionated than I was at the age of five—and I no longer had that abominable walker, which was real progress. I didn't

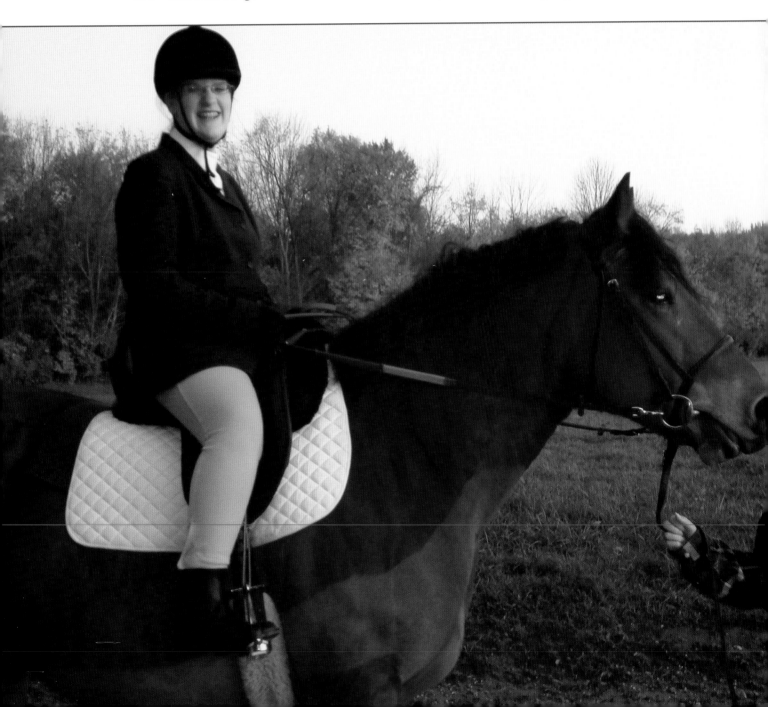

like Western riding at all anymore, and sometimes I just sat on your back, wondering how on earth I ever got on and off of those bulky Western saddles. I was immensely grateful for the more liberating but much more disciplined English saddle. And for you, of course, Clance.

I enjoyed the challenge that both you, Clancy, and the English discipline provided me. Arlene hollering at me to keep my heels out of your sides kept me on my toes. Instinctively, I double-checked the reins to see that they were still at a perfect length. It makes me smile now as I think back.

Quietly, I squeeze your sides and give them a gentle tap with my heels, asking you softly to trot. You take off at a beautiful, even trot, long-paced and steady.

The thing that renders me speechless is your response to my touch—my verbal command to trot is only a low murmur. After awhile I abandoned posting and worked on a sitting trot. You were so amazing. I could now sit through a trot without major issues. We worked on my bouncy hands together, making progress each week. It was a thrill to trot you around the entire arena and trot you through a course for a show that we entered together.

I consider it a miracle that you chose me, Clance.

You taught me more lessons about life than I can recount. One thing I'll always, always love about you is your odd little quirks. It's my firm belief that perfection is not what forms your love for something or someone. No. It's imperfections that make you love unconditionally, in an unexplainable manner. Clancy, you were terrified of the lift and any noises overhead. As a matter of fact, we always had to take care when mounting because you just couldn't stand awkward, strange noises. But you were willing to give me your very best. You gave me your trust.

And, dear Lord, let's not forget those trail rides! You jumped a mile every time a fly bit you. Clance. Baby, I know they hurt when they bite, but was it really the end of the world? I know you nearly threw me from the saddle once, maybe twice, because you did some odd dancing with just your hindquarters. Such behavior frustrated the

◄ Cassey on Clancy

heck out of many other riders, but I just took it all in stride. You were being you, and I couldn't ask more of you when you gave me so much already.

Arlene's telling me to hold you back to a walk now as we trot down the long side of the arena. I silently sit back more, gently giving the reins a pull, asking you to slow down. We round a corner, and I look over to smile at Arlene, reaching out at the same time to pat you on the neck.

Because of you, Clancy, I was the recipient of the 2007 Outstanding Improvement Award at Fieldstone Farm. I never really expected it. We came so far together. Never did I dream that I might lose you.

You always had respiratory issues and such, so you had your good days and bad days. But the actual incident that took your life was due to ongoing hoof problems. I was shocked when I found out that you had been euthanized. You were much too young and had so many more lessons to teach. We won many ribbons together as a team, the majority of them blue. And boy, did I love you.

I realize, Clancy, that you were a fleeting wisp of glory, a precious memory to hold onto for the rest of my life. While I'll always have our show ribbons and memories to remember you by, you will always have a piece of my heart. You changed my life forever.

Rest in peace, big guy.

About Cassey

Cassey is a sixteen-year-old sophomore and honors student in Painesville, Ohio. She lives with her parents, Joe and Shari, and two younger brothers. She's riding a new horse at Fieldstone now named Baby Huey. "I loved him from the start, just as I had Tonka and Clancy. We've come a long way together as a team, and I just adore him. He's responsive, he has his quirks, and he's so fun to be around. I can't wait to see how things go in the new year," she says.

About Fieldstone Farm TRC

Through a special partnership with horses, Fieldstone Farm Therapeutic Riding Center offers programs designed by professionals to foster personal growth and individual achievement for people with disabilities.

TACO:
A COWHORSE WANNABE

— Suzen Jones —

"I just stood there, amazed."

Suzen Jones of Grand View, Idaho, has ridden horses most of her life and knows a good horse when she sees one. Her first memories of horseback riding were sitting in front of her dad on a horse named Pete. In college, she was on a women's equine drill team, but then she sold her horse and didn't ride for several years. She married, had children, and got involved in life's busy activities. Then, like many women who leave behind their horse passion for family responsibilities, she began to feel the need to reconnect with horses when she was older.

So in 2002, Suzen decided to get back into horseback riding. She began to shop around and ended up looking at an athletic sorrel gelding owned by a woman in Boise. He was a pretty boy with a flaxen mane and tail, and Suzen instinctively knew he was the one she wanted. His barn name was Taco. Not only was Taco the perfect size for Suzen—14.2 hands—but his gentle demeanor at just three years old was enough to convince her he was exactly what she was looking for to carry her safely in her middle age. She was not disappointed. She went on a pack trip with Taco shortly after bringing him home. "He was very smart and savvy," Suzen said.

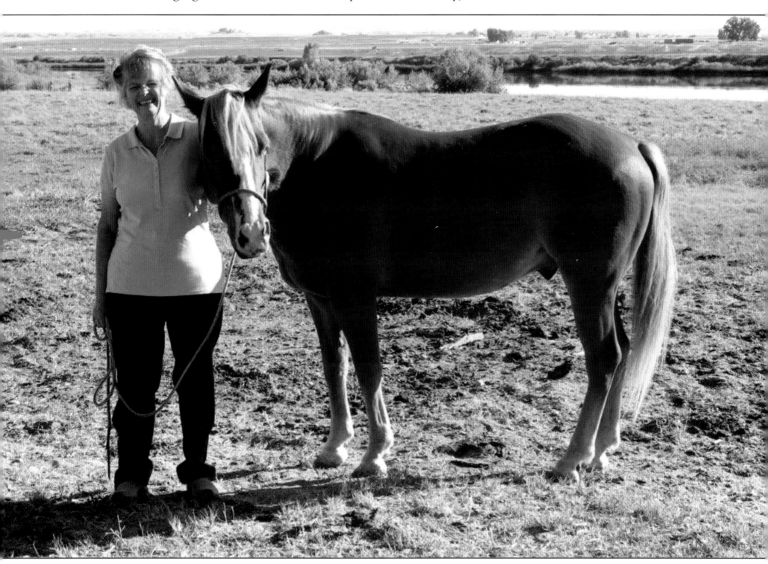

Suzen Jones and Taco

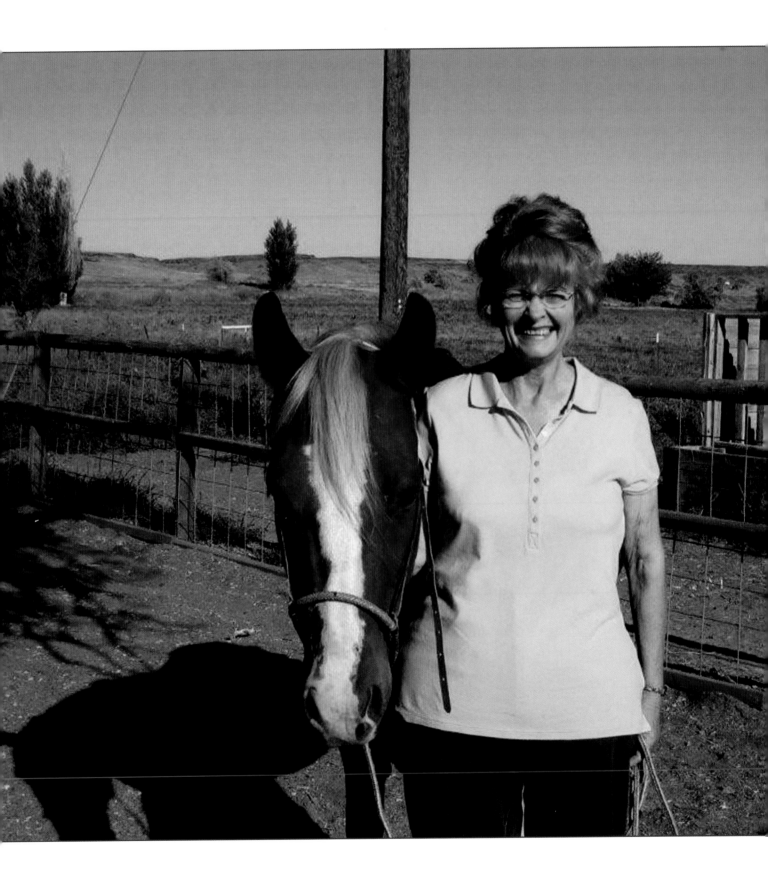

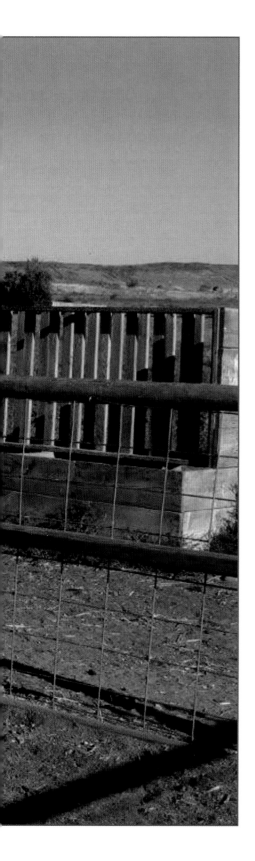

Suzen's husband, Chuck, manages ranch land for J. R. Simplot in southern Idaho and rides the company horses. Their home sits on the cliffs overhanging the Snake River, surrounded by high desert pasture back-dropped by the Owyhee Mountain range. This rugged, beautiful territory is perfect rangeland for herds of cattle, and it is wrangled by a group of cowboys who keep track of the cattle on horseback.

Taco occupied a pasture with a few other horses close to the house for easy access. In the spring, around 125 older Hereford cows and their calves are pastured close to the house until the calves are old enough to be turned out on public land.

Shortly after Suzen bought Taco, she was injured and couldn't ride for several months while she healed. So Chuck kept Taco going; they rounded up cattle as Taco made his way through the rocky landscape, surefooted, calm, and reliable. Suzen didn't realize the depth of all that Taco learned during those months out on the range. She did know, however, that Taco had good cowhorse breeding. His registered name was Teponita San Sport, which told her that he was from the lineage of the well-bred and famous cutting horse Peppy San Badger. When she checked his credentials, she found Peppy's name in Taco's lineage. But she didn't fully appreciate his cowhorse lineage until the day his speed and genetic know-how saved her from danger.

It was early morning, and Suzen had gone out to the paddock to let the horses into the big pasture to graze on the scrubby desert grasslands. Not paying much attention, Suzen didn't notice that some of the cattle were also in the big pasture. It was early spring. The cattle had recently dropped their calves—and ranchers needed to take careful precautions around the new mothers, who defended their calves with fury. These range cows could be defensive, aggressive, and dangerous with their calves close by—something Suzen had nearly forgotten that morning.

And this morning she failed to notice the cow—its head up, charging at her—until it was too late to get out of the way.

"Chuck had always told me that when you see a cow's head up like that, you'd better run," she said. "I guess that the brown cow had hidden its calf somewhere nearby—but I never saw it."

Suzen had been standing by the gate as the horses walked single file through from the paddock out into the bigger pasture. Taco was last in line. About the time the first horse got past her, she suddenly looked up and saw the cow charging.

Plans for escape flashed through her head. "Should I jump up on the fence, or should I just run and hope I'm faster than the cow?" she thought. Knowing that neither option was fool-proof, she began to panic. In a flash, she understood the gravity of her situation and began to turn away, to somehow lessen the impact of the inevitable.

But she barely had time to react when she saw a red streak flash past her. She spun around and saw the most amazing thing. Sensing Suzen's danger, Taco had run to head off the angry cow. Ears flat, head down, he met the cow head on and steered it away from Suzen and back out into the scabland, as if that's what he was meant to do.

"I didn't even realize how cowy he was until then," said Suzen, even though he'd spent hours rounding up cattle on the ranch.

"He even bit the cow on the butt a few times," she laughed. "I just stood there, amazed. When he got the cow far enough away, he put his head down and continued to graze as if nothing happened. I'll never forget that."

Taco has turned out to be one of the best horses Suzen ever owned. Not only does he willingly do anything he's asked, he's gentle and calm with Suzen and Chuck's grandsons.

"He's the perfect horse," said Suzen. "He's a little cowhorse wannabe."

AFTER VIETNAM

— Dave Morgan —

"I can have the worst day of my life, walk out and talk to my horses, and everything is suddenly okay."

Since Vietnam, Americans have learned how to better care for and appreciate veterans of war. Those who come home wounded and hurting now have a new source for therapy: the Horses for Heroes Program. The North American Riding for the Handicapped Association has developed this program aimed at helping wounded service personnel tap into the healing power of horses. Although the program is still new, many wounded soldiers have been able to realize the physical and emotional power of hippotherapy.

But for Vietnam War veteran Dave Morgan, the program only verifies what he already knows: that horses have amazing therapeutic capabilities. He also knows that not all war scars are physical. Some of the most severe are those unseen wounds that fester deep inside the soul. Dave's wounds are never far from the surface. His story began long before the Horses for Heroes program—back in 1967 when he came home from combat in Vietnam with severe post-traumatic stress disorder.

"I don't talk about my time in Vietnam because some things are best left unsaid," Dave says. "Suffice it to say my horses are the main thing that has kept me sane since I came home more than forty years ago."

Dave grew up in El Paso, Texas, around horses. His father managed a horse ranch for a while and a couple of dairies. Young Dave was always around livestock, which is what kept him interested in horses over the years.

But growing up wasn't easy for him.

"I got into a lot of trouble in El Paso. When I was seventeen years old, the judge gave me the option of either going into the military or spending six years in jail," said Dave. "I chose the navy. That's the way things were back in the sixties. Many troubled teens were given the military as an ultimatum. For me, the military was the biggest wake-up call I had in my life. I wouldn't trade my military time for the world, and

Dave Morgan with Lukachukai ➤

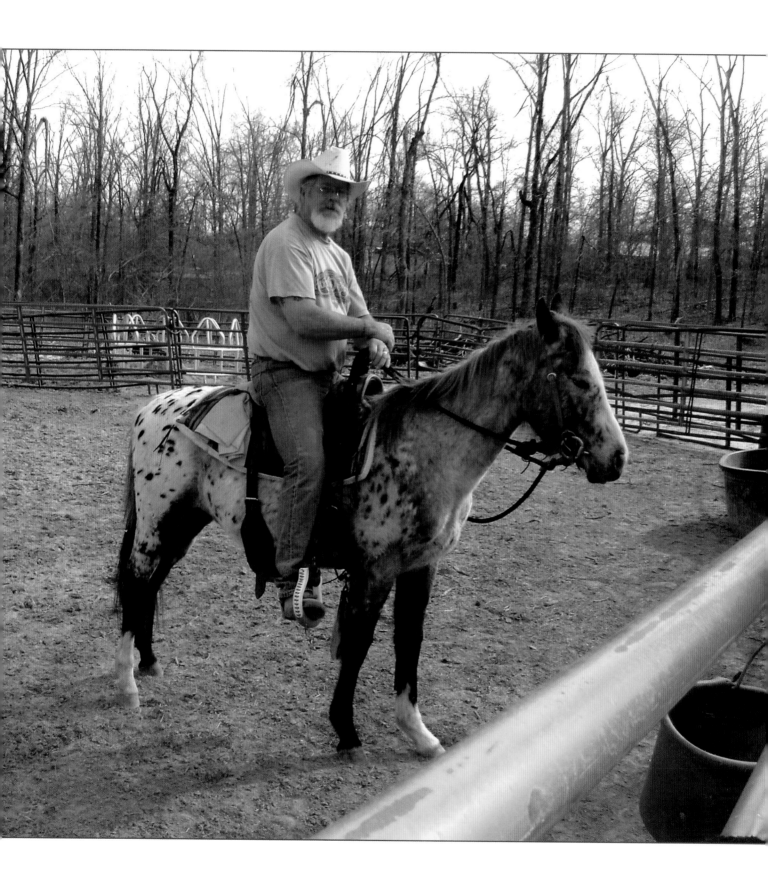

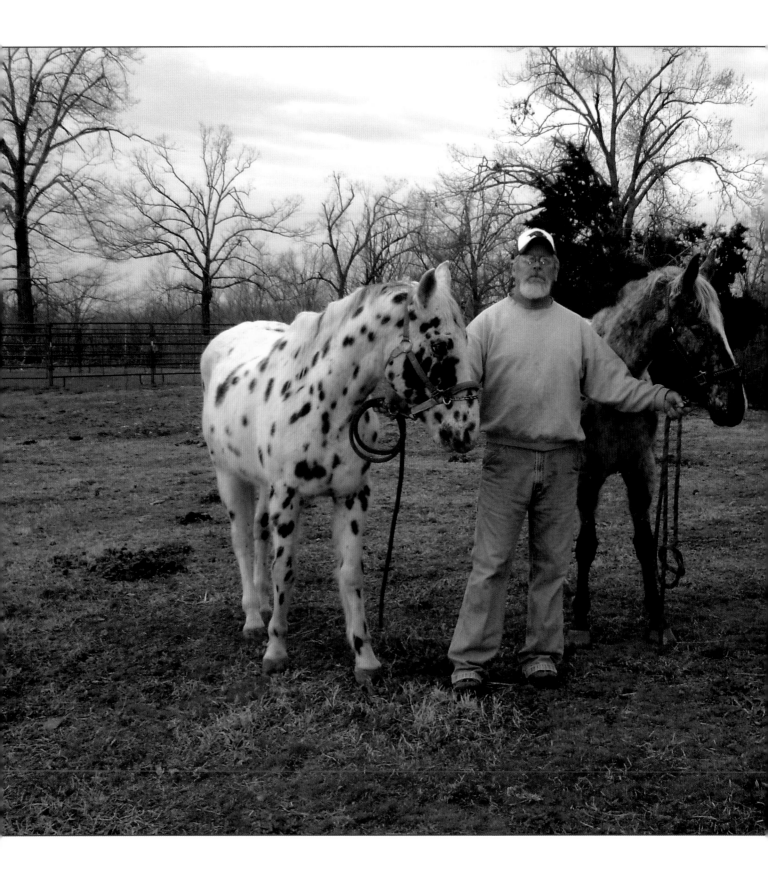

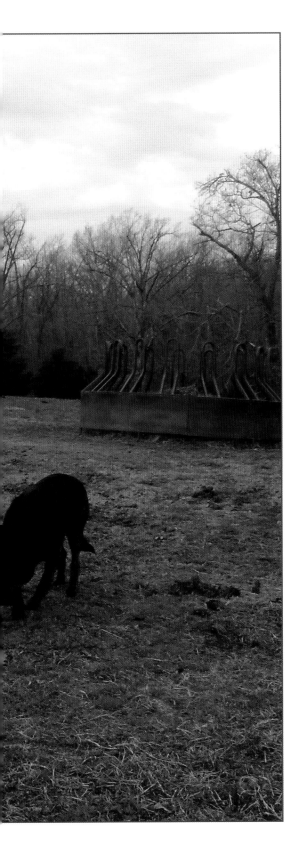

I'm grateful for it because it got me on track with my life. But I wouldn't want to do it again, and I wouldn't wish it on anyone else."

The navy straightened Dave up. He was out on a ship for one tour and on the ground for two. He got out of the military, scarred but functional, when he was twenty-one, and he bummed around for a bit and then went to work at the El Paso Airport. From El Paso, he moved to Casper, Wyoming, for a couple of years and then started working for Exxon in uranium. After many, many years in the mining business for Exxon, Dave retired early.

While his life may sound somewhat ordinary, his emotional survival since returning from Vietnam is not. Post-traumatic stress disorder is an anxiety disorder that can develop after exposure to a terrifying event or ordeal in which grave physical harm occurred or was threatened. People with PTSD have persistent frightening thoughts from memories of their ordeal. They often feel emotionally numb, experience sleep problems, and can be easily startled. War veterans with PTSD often feel deeply angry and stressed out. Dave's symptoms drove him to the one source he knew could help—his horses.

"Over the years, my horses have kept me sane," he says. "They keep my head clear. I take medication to help me sleep and to keep my temper from flaring

◄ Dave Morgan and his horses King and Snowflake

and the nightmares at bay. But I can have the worst day of my life, walk out and talk to my horses, and everything is suddenly okay. They have been the best therapy money could buy."

Not only have horses been therapy for Dave, they've been part of his livelihood.

After living in Gillette, Wyoming for several years, Dave and his wife bought the town of Belle, Wyoming, in the northeast corner of the state in 1992. The town of Belle had been incorporated in 1913 and closed down in 1917. They named their horse ranch The Belle Wyoming Ranch. In their second year there, they started breeding Appaloosas, using the stallion Winnie's Golden King as their foundation sire. "We had up to twenty horses at a time there. It was beautiful. I also had three Mustangs—I had bought two at a prison where the inmates trained them, and the other I bought from the Bureau of Land Management training station, where I also learned how to train them," said Dave.

But eventually the winters in Wyoming became too much because of arthritis in Dave's hands, so he decided to move to a warmer climate in Arizona.

"We put the horses up for sale and left Wyoming with just two: an Appaloosa stallion and a Quarter Horse mare," said Dave. "These two horses were the foundation of my next herd."

While in Arizona, Dave became even more involved in horses. He became involved in horse rescue in Scottsdale and bought a couple of Thoroughbred stallions and a mare

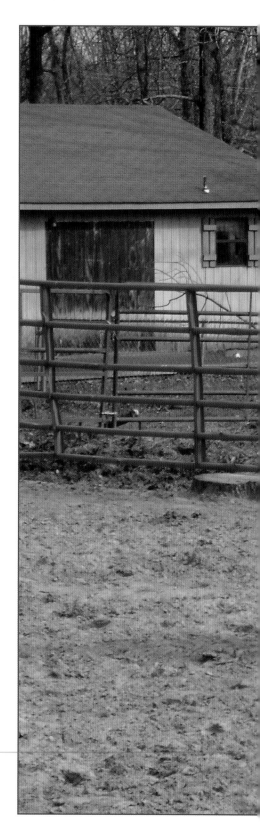

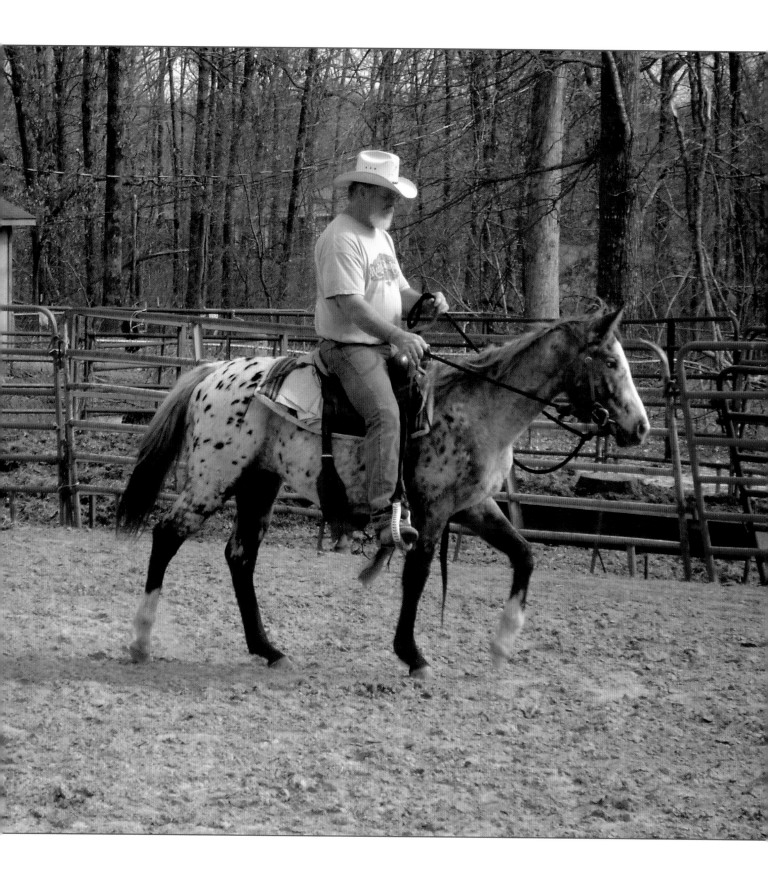

and colt. From there, he bought several more Thoroughbreds right off the racetrack. This was the beginning of a great breeding adventure.

"They were fantastic horses," said Dave. "Two of my Thoroughbreds, Odds On and Merchant Prince, had raced four times and placed first twice. When Odds On was

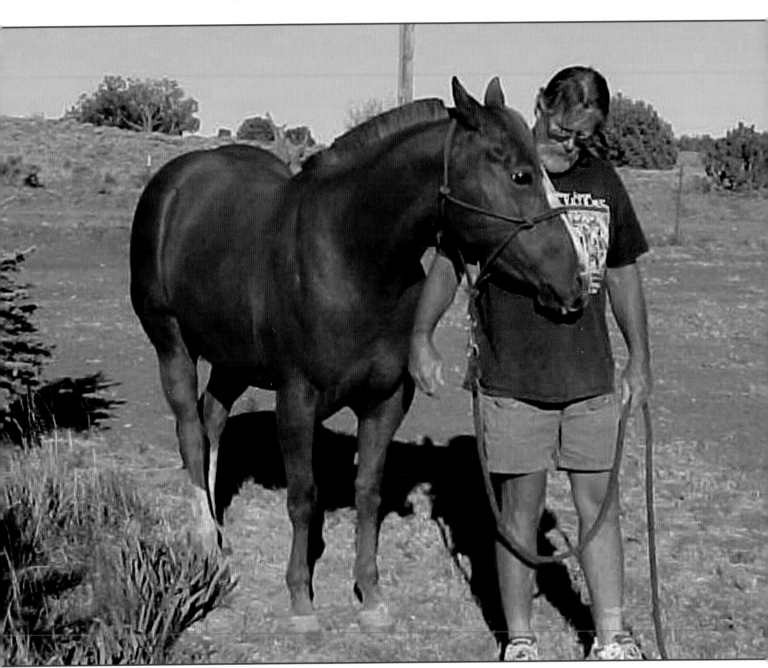

Dave Morgan with Midgen De Royale

sold as a yearling, he went for $375,000. I bought both horses for $2,500." Dave crossed the Thoroughbred racehorses with his Appaloosa mares and liked what he got.

After a few years, the Arizona climate got to the Morgans, so they packed up and moved to Arkansas, where they are now retired. Winters are mild there, and it stays green year round. Before moving, they sold all their horses except the Appaloosas.

"The truth is, Appaloosas have to be the best listeners in the horse world," said Dave. "We love sitting on the back porch in the morning enjoying a coffee and watching the spots in the pasture."

Forty years of horse therapy has helped scar over and soothe Dave's memories of Vietnam. Without horses, he's not sure how his life would have gone.

"Horses keep me on a relatively even keel," said Dave. "I can have the worst day possible—be ready to kill everyone in my path and myself—but an hour or so with my horses soothes everything over and I'm okay. My horses and my dog return love and respect and are fantastic listeners. I can talk to them, say whatever I want or need, and they listen without interrupting."

FROSTED CHEROKEE

—— Cheryl Farrens ——

"Panic gripped me when

I realized the seriousness of the situation."

I grew up in a suburb near Rochester, New York, and even though I didn't own a horse, every year my dad would bring home a little collectible Breyer horse for me. As my collection grew over time, so did my love for horses.

My dad was raised on a farm in Virginia, and whenever our family would go back to visit them, I begged to get up on one of the big plow horses and ride around. Soon my horse love turned into a full-blown addiction, and I knew that horse statues wouldn't be enough for me. So, after much prodding and begging, I convinced my parents to let me take horseback riding lessons, where I finally learned the nuts and bolts of how to ride a real horse. Over the years, I became an accomplished rider.

Finally, when I was in high school, I asked my parents if I could buy a horse as long as I could pay for boarding costs. They said yes.

Is that all I ever had to do? I thought to myself.

So I bought a Quarter Horse and used her for hunter jumper events. She served me well through my high school years. When I went off to college, my dad, who was then in his fifties, kept her and rode her. When I got married and moved to Texas, I gave her to a racetrack to use as a pony for the racehorses.

Eventually Dad retired and moved down to Texas to be near me, since I was an only child. My husband and I had built a house on some land near Dallas and put up a pen

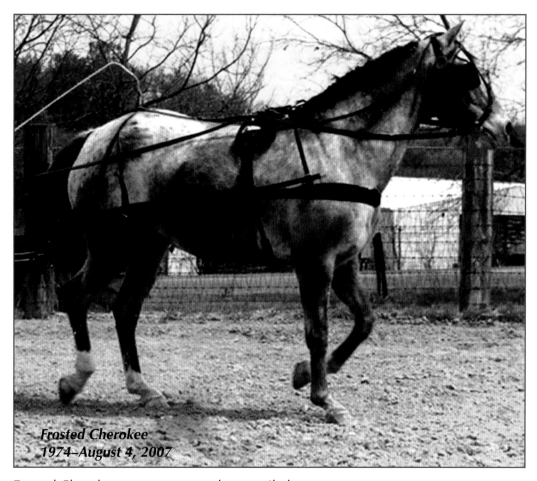

Frosted Cherokee
1974–August 4, 2007

Frosted Cherokee was an extremely versatile horse.

for horses. I bought a part-Thoroughbred Palomino, and Dad and I took turns riding her. But that got old pretty fast because we both wanted to ride. It was clear we needed another horse.

One day the man I bought the Palomino from introduced me to Frosted Cherokee. That little Appaloosa mare could do anything. She was very, very careful with novice riders, but with experienced riders, she would really test them until they proved they could handle her spirit.

Frosted Cherokee was one of those mares that could do anything you asked. Her versatility was amazing. She worked cows, was a great babysitter and a champion driver, and very smart. She was my lesson horse until she was more than thirty years old. She got herself into some situations throughout her life that would have probably killed any other horse, but Cherokee always waited patiently for us to come and find her and take her home.

I used to loan her out to cutters, and she was also a champion barrel horse. When I had a couple of students who wanted to barrel race, I used her for that. Several cowboys wanted to buy her when she was twenty-six because she could cut a cow like crazy. They also used her for team penning. We used her as a parade horse and as a cart horse. We used her for driving and doing performances and giving driving lessons. The gentleman who taught me how to drive gave some demonstrations on television with her, so she's also a TV star.

You could hardly overwork Cherokee—she had a lot go give—but if she did get tired, she'd stop and look back at the rider as if to say, "We're done *now*!"

I broke her to drive. When she'd had enough driving, she'd stop, back the cart up, and turn the wheels until they'd stop right at the ditch. She'd look over her shoulder at me as if to say, "Okay, we're done now, right?" She never tipped the cart, but she made it very clear that we were done.

Did I say that Frosted Cherokee could do anything?

Even though Cherokee had numerous talents and accomplishments, I will never forget the day she saved my dad's life. That day showed me the true spirit and intellect of this very special horse.

It was a cool fall afternoon when my father, who was then seventy-four years old, decided to go on a horseback ride out across the fallow fields. Dad mounted Cherokee, I rode the Palomino, and my friend Kathy, who was boarding her Thoroughbred at our place, mounted up to go along. We rode out across the fields—a ride we'd been on dozens of times before, and we were all relaxed and enjoying the ride and the fabulous fall colors.

But that all changed when Dad decided he wanted to race.

He took off at a full run on Cherokee. Kathy and I were on Thoroughbreds, but it was still a job trying to catch up to Dad on Cherokee. We were running full-guns, and I remember hearing Dad laughing. Suddenly I saw something fly from Cherokee. It wasn't my dad—it was one of his stirrups. Panic gripped me when I realized the seriousness of the situation. Without both stirrups for balance, Dad began to sway dangerously in the saddle. Then, trying to keep his balance, he lost his reins as well. He held onto the saddle horn but was swaying dangerously in the saddle at a full gallop.

Cherokee instantly knew something was wrong and made some adjustments to help Dad regain his balance. Instead of going into a panic, like some horses might do, she very carefully slowed down and came to a very gentle stop. Then she turned her head around to check and see that Dad was okay. Although he was a bit shaken, he was still laughing. Cherokee, on her own, turned around and walked back to where the stirrup was, under a tree. She knew exactly what had happened and exactly what my dad needed.

Eventually I sold the farm and gave Cherokee to the family who bought it. I moved up to Maryland, but I went back about a year and a half later to see my good friend Cherokee. When I saw her in the front yard, I felt sick. She was a skeleton. Her new owners obviously weren't feeding her. I knew if I called the sheriff right away, they'd put her down because she was so old. So I told the people, "You either give me that horse back, or I'll call the sheriff."

So they let me take her back. I boarded her for about six months with a friend of my trainers in Texas until she put on enough weight to ship her up to Maryland, where I had moved. Then I put her out to pasture for the rest of her life. She deserved a life of ease after all she'd given my dad and me.

Last summer when Cherokee was thirty-four years old, I came outside and saw that she had been rolling in the night. I could tell she was in trouble. The vet came out and gave her some painkillers, and then we led her out into the back field. She staggered a little, lay down, and was gone.

Frosted Cherokee was the most amazing, versatile, intuitive horse I've ever owned. Not only could she do just about anything, she was there when my dad needed her the most. I still think back on that day in amazement, and I realize that because of Cherokee's intuitive nature, she was able to save my dad from harm. She will always be a part of my fondest horse memories.

A HORSE NAMED BEN

— *Stanzi Miller* —

"Then in my second year I met Ben, a partially sighted Suffolk Punch gelding. Little did I know when I met him that Ben would become the horse that would make such a difference in my life."

"**M**iss Miller," my rheumatologist said, "you have fibromyalgia."

Her words echoed in my mind. Finally, I thought, there is a name for this muscle stiffness, relentless fatigue, and pain. Her diagnosis explained everything. My doctor went on to stay, "We believe your symptoms were brought on by that fall you took when you were nineteen years old."

Fibromyalgia presents with chronic, widespread pain. While symptoms vary from person to person and from day to day, there are times when flares can leave a person reeling from intense pain, blurred vision, and any number of problems.

My mind flashed back to the day of the accident that brought me to this place. Being a horse fanatic, I had enrolled in a hunt seat class in college. Everything went well until I went on a hack. I got bucked off as the horse changed gaits from a trot to a canter. I spent three months recovering from a cervical neck injury, broken arm, and concussion. As soon as I recovered, I went right back to riding horses—but I couldn't quite get over my fear of falling.

Twenty years later, little did I realize my fall in college would result in this devastating syndrome called fibromyalgia. Neither could I imagine that another horse—a therapy horse named Ben—would come to my rescue in so many ways.

Fibromyalgia changed my life incrementally over time. I was forced to give up my job and sports. Fatigue, muscle stiffness, and pain became my constant companions. As the years went by, walking became impossible. The "Fibro Thief" prevailed, taking away any of my career aspirations after college. I mourned my former life of strength and happiness.

To help with all the symptoms of the illness, my doctor suggested that I find some type of exercise I could do. I started thinking of how great it would be to hear that soft nicker again. I longed to feel as alive and happy as I had been when I rode a horse in college. So I decided to apply to be a client at Hoofbeats Therapeutic Riding Center in Lexington, Virginia.

I rode several horses my first year at Hoofbeats as an independent rider and even won the Division Championship. Then in my second year I met Ben, a partially sighted Suffolk Punch gelding. Little

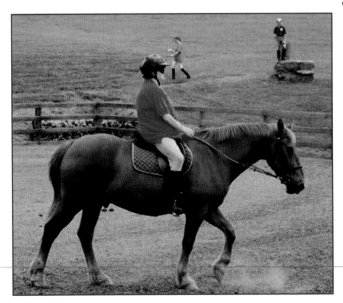

Constance Stanzi riding Ben

did I know when I met him that Ben would become the horse that would make such a difference in my life.

The first day we met, he did something very special for me. After our first lesson we stopped next to the mounting block near the barn, and my ground crew arrived to assist me in dismounting. It took several people to help me get on and off a horse. As I attempted to dismount, I ran into problems because the muscles in my legs are tight and stiff. As hard as I tried, I could not stretch my legs to make the distance between the block and Ben.

"I don't think Ben can get any closer to the block," said Maria, the assistant instructor.

"But I can't reach the block with my foot," I said, wondering how I was going to get out of this predicament.

But Ben knew. Sensing my problem, suddenly Ben decided he would shove himself into the mounting block without any of us asking him to, making it possible for me to dismount.

The ground crew exploded with emotion. Ben knew exactly what the problem was and went that extra mile to help me—all on his own. It floored me to think Ben caused himself discomfort just so I could dismount. This little incident told me so much about Ben. He did numerous remarkable things for me that year.

But even after riding for more than a year, I continued to have significant fears. The trip from the barn to the riding ring involved traveling down a long hill. A few times I got flustered when we started going too fast. I became fearful, thinking I might fall. I got so scared that I braced. Ben sometimes fretted when I got scared. A few times he even stumbled, but I stayed on him.

Carol, my dressage instructor said, "See? You didn't fall. You conquered your fears." I didn't feel that I had overcome anything at that point. The possibility of falling terrified me even more. I saw myself falling and falling and falling. I wondered how I would ever be able to fix this feeling of terror.

Carol suggested some interesting methods for dealing with this fear. Besides using a neoprene saddle attachment to make me feel secure, she suggested that I count out loud from one to ten as I traveled down the hill, stopping each time at ten. As I chanted each number, I halted at ten to regain my balance. If I forget to say ten, Ben stopped regardless.

Ben and I prepared for the fall show at the Horse Center, which Ben hated. For some reason, his calm demeanor turned into wild-eyed spookiness. I did my best to help him relax, but nothing worked. It's funny, but his fear reminded me of my own fears. But now it was my turn to be the calm one as we entered the show ring.

I trusted Ben so implicitly that I rode him without fear with a relaxed, balanced, and centered seat in both my dressage test, and my dressage freestyle musical event. We zigzagged all around that arena in a nervous, jiggy quick walk. I got so turned around during our test after a wild-eyed terrified Ben went the wrong way during the freestyle event that I forgot what we were supposed to do next. In a split second, I made up the rest of our routine. We came in second place, with a higher score for freestyle compared to the dressage test.

After we were finished, I realized what a team Ben and I were. We both had our fears and weaknesses, but together we were strong.

Ben gave me the gift of freedom and helped me forget about my disability. He became my legs. He helped me forget about fear. With all the ways he showed love toward me, he healed me from the effects of the accident. Because of him, today I am free.

About Stanzi

I enjoy dressage competition, writing fantasy fiction, and moderating the Jericho Rally Point. I love to spend time with my border collie. Ben couldn't adjust when Hoofbeats moved to the Virginia Horse Center in 2007, so he is now the star at Equi-kids Therapeutic Riding Center in Virginia Beach.

FREEDOM FOR MIA

— *Brian and Teresa Bester* —

"My legs feel free when I ride."

When Brian and Teresa Bester of Bainbridge Township, Ohio, found out they were expecting their third child in 1999, they were thrilled. Already the parents of two boys, they were fully in tune with the rigors of parenthood and anticipated the arrival of child number three.

When Mia finally arrived, with her big brown eyes and apparent perfect health, the family rejoiced. *Finally—another female in the house*, thought Teresa. They had no way of seeing into the future, and no reason to suspect that Mia had any problems.

But when Mia turned ten months old, Teresa started noticing that the baby wasn't reaching the typical developmental benchmarks she should. She couldn't even sit up

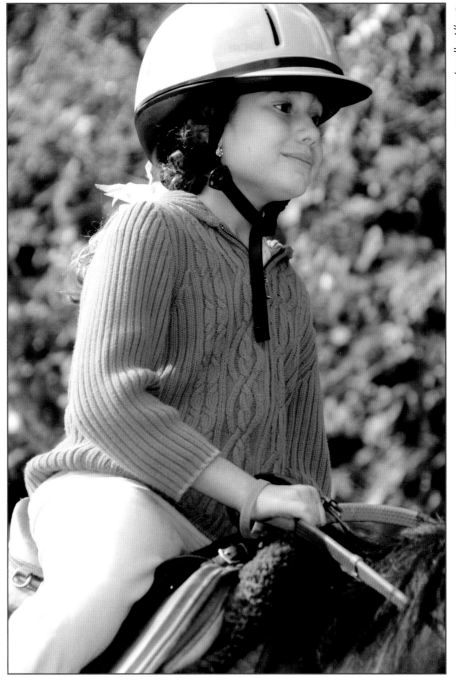

PHOTO BY *Janelle Alberts*

yet—and Teresa's fears began to grow. As a pediatric nurse, she knew something was not right.

"She would never lay flat on her back, and I never saw the palms of her hands," said Teresa. "To clean her hands, I always had to unclench her fists."

So Teresa contacted a neurologist, who ran a battery of tests—including a CAT scan. The tests revealed that Mia had too much white matter in her brain, which is a symptom consistent with cerebral palsy.

This is not what Brian and Teresa had envisioned for their little girl. Doctors diagnosed Mia with spastic diplegia, a form of cerebral palsy that affects her lower extremities. Because her leg muscles were so stiff, doctors said Mia would spend her life in a wheelchair and never have bowel or bladder control or be able to walk.

The Besters struggled to get a grip on their new reality, but they were not ready to settle for the doctors' prognosis. So instead of focusing on what the doctors said Mia would never do, Brian and Teresa focused on letting Mia set her own limitations.

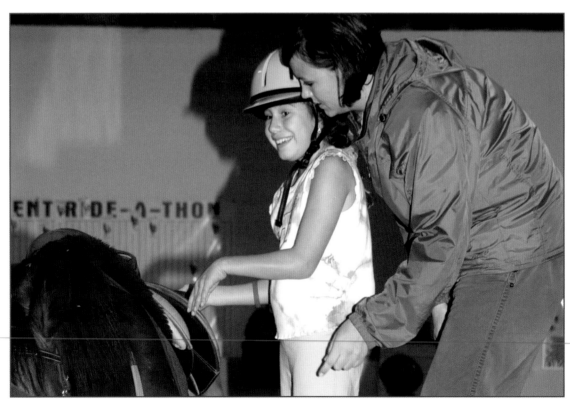

PHOTO BY *Janelle Alberts*

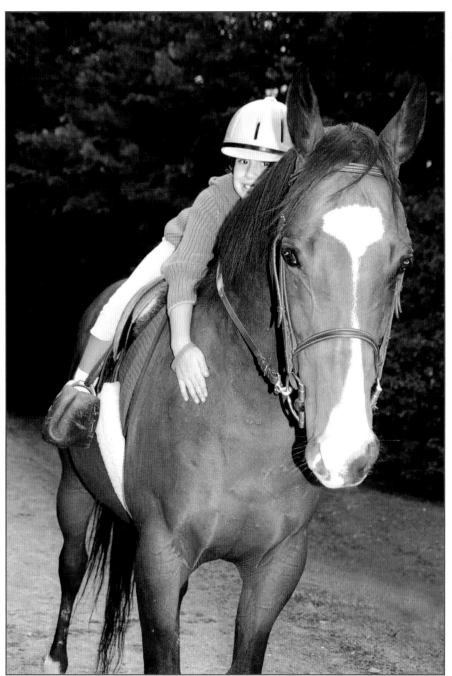

PHOTO BY *Janelle Alberts*

Not far from where the Besters lived was a therapeutic riding center. Teresa had always known about the place and had often hoped one of her sons would volunteer there one day. When Mia was just two years old, Teresa gave them a call, convinced that Mia would be a great candidate. She was not only smart and had great verbal skills, but she knew how to take directions well too. Her verbal skills were so good because she had to tell her family what she wanted—she couldn't get things herself.

"I asked the center if they would please give it a try with Mia, even though she was only two years old, just to see if she could do it," said Teresa, even though she admitted she didn't have full confidence the program would help her daughter physically. "I thought she would have fun," Teresa said.

But two months after Mia started her weekly forty-five-minute hippotherapy sessions, she crawled for the first time. "She used to bunny-hop all over the house instead of crawling," said Teresa. "It was the rhythmic motion of the horse—one hip in front of the other—that helped her crawl." Before long, Mia was pulling herself up into a standing position, and then she was using a walker to get around the house. Mia became stronger than anyone predicted.

"The first time I watched Mia ride, I was in tears," said Teresa. "She looked so fluid. I could imagine how she felt, being so uninhibited. She doesn't have to worry about where to put her legs or what muscle is pulling in the wrong direction. She has freedom."

Mia has her own sentiments about horseback riding. She says, "I don't have to hear my therapist or my mom say, 'Don't drag your foot!'"

Riding a horse requires good strength and motor skills. Mia uses her thigh muscles to grip the horse; to hold herself upright, she uses her core, shoulder, and neck muscles. Her hand muscles hold the reins. But she gets as much joy from being on a horse as she does the physical benefits of riding horses.

"My legs feel free when I ride," said Mia. Riding makes her forget about all the work she's doing. On horseback, she's uninhibited and filled with an indescribable joy.

Mia's favorite horse was Latte. He was so in tune with her movements that all she had to do was say "Trot," and Latte would take off. The horses at the therapeutic riding center are trained to stop when they feel a rider lean forward. They think this motion is a sign that a rider is falling off. But Mia has to lean forward to bring her heels back for a trot, so Latte learned—just for Mia—the verbal cues.

Latte broke her leg one day, and Mia did not see her for months during the horse's rehabilitation. On one of Mia's riding days, Latte was being led across a parking lot as Mia was walking into the center. "Latte realized it was Mia and took off on her hurt leg toward Mia, then came up and gave her a nudge. It was like two long-lost friends reunited," said Teresa.

Mary Goff Hipp, senior riding instructor at Fieldstone Farm Therapeutic Riding Center where Mia rides, says that she's watched the most amazing growth in Mia over the last seven years. "This child is so incredibly motivated. She wants to do exercises at home to make herself a better rider. There is something intrinsic with this child that gives her such a huge heart. In class she's always saying 'Good job' to the other riders."

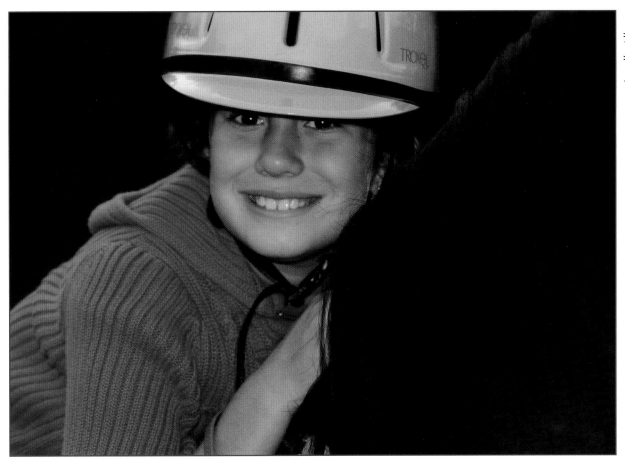

PHOTO BY *Janelle Alberts*

There are also students at Fieldstone who have cognitive disabilities. One day a new student with a cognitive disability asked Mia why she needed a cane. Mia answered, "I need it to help me walk because I can't walk as good as you."

The little girl answered, "I'm sorry."

"This interaction was so precious," said Mary. "Mia is so kind and so understanding with the other children—she truly is amazing."

Mia is now a confident nine-year-old. Over the years, she's become an accomplished rider, winning ribbons at horse shows and making her family proud. She's also a third-grader. She tossed away the walker years ago and now walks with and sometimes without the assistance of a cane. But she still feels the most confident on the back of a horse.

Mia's two brothers both play sports. Mia also participates in ballet, using her cane as an extension of her arm. She also played T-ball, using her cane to hit the ball. Horseback riding gives Mia the chance to participate in something different than her brothers, and they love watching their sister ride. "Her disability has exposed them to a variety of people with disabilities, and they've learned not to be judgmental and to have kinder hearts," said Teresa.

The riding center hosts three horse shows a year. In 2005, Mia was named student of the year. In 2007, she scored the most high points in horse shows, and in 2008, she was student of the month. Mia's story was also featured in the September 2007 edition of *Parents* magazine.

RAIN

— Kay Loy —

*"If you want something different in life,
you have to do something different."*

My life spiraled out of control. Nightmares, or, even worse, insomnia left me exhausted and unable to function. I had lapses in memory. Sometimes I'd wake up in a different location or not even know where I was. I also had unexplained panic attacks that left me frozen in fear.

I was diagnosed with brain injury, depression, and post-traumatic stress disorder. Treatment followed: individual counseling, group counseling, and, of course, medication. I didn't think anyone would understand the devastating affects of spousal abuse, so I withdrew.

I grew up in the Illinois Valley. Five miles from our home was a riding stable, and it was my life's mission from the time I was five years old to get my parents to take me there. Finally, when I was seven years old, I began lessons, and I continued riding every chance I had until I was fourteen years old—enough time for horses to make an indelible impression on my mind.

Life went on, and I eventually joined the army as a chaplain's assistant. I was stationed in Fort Lewis, Washington, and in northern Germany during my eight years in the military. I was released in 1985, but I stayed in Europe because I was married to another American in the military. I was able to get a job there with the Federal Service System.

While we were stationed at Fort Irwin, California, I was able to earn an associate's degree in general business and got another job with the Federal System, this time in finance, keeping track of a huge military budget. After my spouse's retirement, we moved to Washington State.

When my marriage fell apart a few years later, I turned to the Veteran's

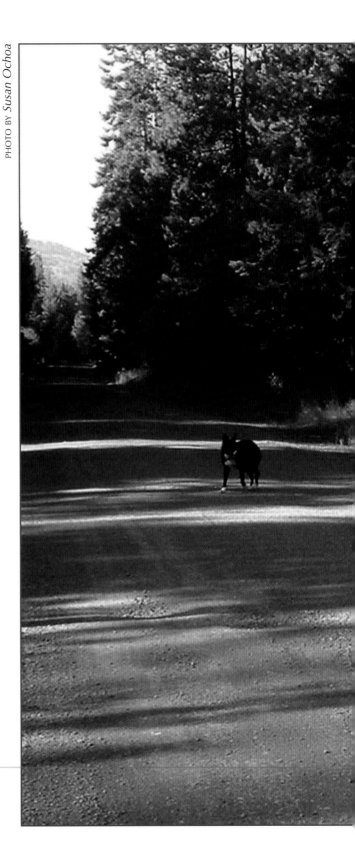

PHOTO BY *Susan Ochoa*

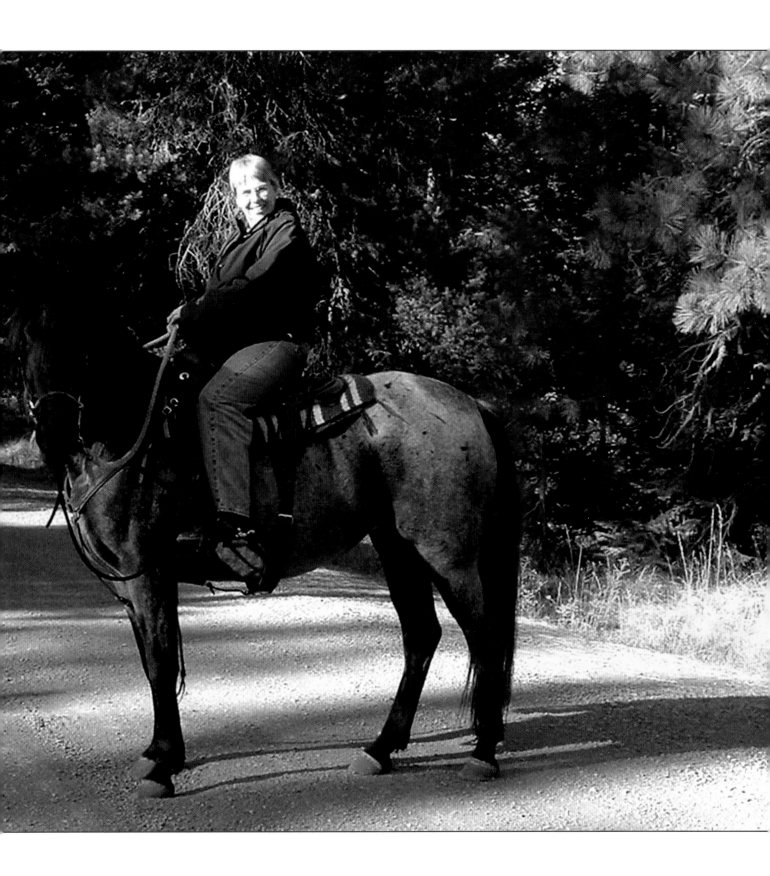

Administration for help. I saw a counselor for many years, but I always felt uncomfortable opening up. My deep fears, anger, and nervousness made me feel like a nutcase at times. My life was out of control, and I didn't know what was wrong. But soon came my diagnosis—a result of severe spousal abuse. My former husband had been an officer in the military.

In 2008, I learned about the Veteran's Administration Horses for Heroes Program through Boots 'n Breeches, a horse therapy facility in Washington State. At the time, I didn't really think it would be therapeutic, but I knew the program would bring back some happy childhood memories of horseback riding. Before I drove up for my first session, the PTSD kicked in, and I became terrified. As a matter of fact, I planned to go there and just tell them I couldn't go through with it.

I was immediately introduced to a horse named Tiger, and the magic began. I couldn't stop thinking about Tiger as I drove home. After that, to help myself get adjusted to the new environment at the therapeutic riding center, I would play with my service dog before my sessions began. This helped me relax and become accustomed to the new environment. I didn't realize how important this was until later in the program as I began to heal.

The program was eight weeks long. Other disabled veterans participate in different programs. I believe we were all impacted differently, depending on our injuries. Some veterans focus on regaining muscle strength and balance, while my problems were the internal, psychological kind.

I rode two horses while I was in therapy: Tiger and Jackie O. I quickly realized that with horses, my connection was far different than with my human counselors. I came to that powerful realization the day I entered the barn in a horrible state of mind. My horse was responding to me differently, and I realized that this big animal could hurt me. It helped me get in touch with my feelings. This horse was reflecting how I felt, unlike human counselors who asked, "How do you feel?" I learned that I needed to connect with my own feelings and take them back under my control. Each time I went to work with the horses after that, I strived to control my emotions and reconnect with the horses. This was the beginning of relearning to live in the moment and escape the dissociative state common with PTSD. This was powerful therapy.

Toward the end of my eight-week horse therapy session, I started asking questions about horse ownership. I decided that I was not going to live without my intuitive horse therapist! I went online to Dreamhorse.com and started my search. I knew what I wanted: a horse five to fifteen years old, good with dogs, within a hundred miles from home, and about a level two. I wrote the names of the horses down as I dreamt of which one would be my new friend and therapist. The last name on my list was "Rain," a beautiful blue roan Tennessee Walker. Deep down I felt like this was the one. I went back and looked again. She was a three-year-old filly and lived seven hundred miles away. But in spite of my criteria, something told me to go get her.

Traveling to look at Rain took me way out of my comfort zone. When I got there, however, the couple, Susan and Louis Ochoa, quickly put me at ease. They offered to let me stay at their home, which was difficult for me to contemplate. But our Christian connection and faith quickly dissolved my fears. I told them that I had very little experience with horses, so they took me on some trail rides like I'd never been before. They gave me a real workout to make sure that I was right for their horse.

At the end of two days, they sat down and asked me if I still wanted the horse. I said, "You don't understand. I came here to buy the horse—that was never a question." The following weekend they loaded Rain and delivered her to a boarding stable.

Boarding Rain wasn't exactly what I wanted. Within two months I made another difficult decision: to sell the city house I had lived in since my divorce. Deep inside I knew this house was destructive to my well-being. It held terrible memories. Selling the house and putting that chapter of my life behind me was a big step in my healing process. I was able purchase a small home with ten acres—enough space for Rain. Since then, my life has been completely different.

I spend time with Rain every day, even if I don't ride. Some days I just brush her out and enjoy her company. The other day I introduced her to a bit. Everything I do with Rain is therapy for me. She allows me to see myself for who I truly am and to regain control of some of my life.

As I watched other veterans in therapy and saw the smiles on their faces, I was deeply moved by their challenges and accomplishments. I know that horses have the ability to take them far. I know Rain has done that for me. I'm so grateful that I decided to be proactive and make a change. After all, if you want something different in your life, you have to do something different.

THE THIEF

— *Ivy Christian* —

"After all I had done to prevent the illness, there it was. . . .
I spent months feeling guilty."

I grew up on a little farm outside of Pullman, Washington. My mother carried me on a horse through a good part of her pregnancy and had me on one soon after I was born. When I was three years old, I got my first pony. Pixie was a black and white dream. For years it seemed as if we were the perfect family, even though my little brother and I fought all the time.

Horses were an important part of our family's life. Both my parents had ridden horses growing up, and my father trained colts for extra income. Mom showed her horse at the local fair in high school, and when she was sixteen years old, she was invited to work on a Tennessee Walker ranch to train horses. She and Grandma had gone there to look at horses to buy when the owner realized that my mother had real talent with horses. But Grandma said no—she needed to come back home and finish high school. So she did.

When I was twelve years old, legendary horse trainer Monty Foreman came to the Pullman area for the very first time, and my mother attended the clinic. Foreman taught his audience new things, like riding on diagonals, posting at a trot, and lead changes. People who attended the clinics were amazed that horses could actually work better knowing these techniques.

Mom came home from the clinic and taught me how to do all these things on Pixie. Before long I was doing sliding stops and rollbacks on him. During this time,

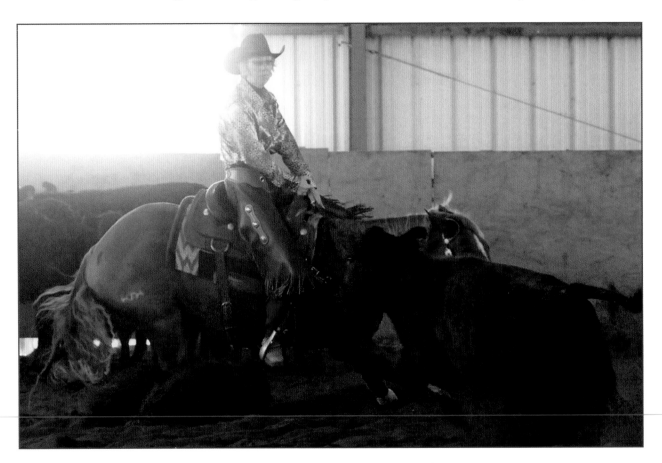

Ivy cutting on Jerry

my parents were also involved in the cutting sport, and Dad owned a double-bred Hancock horse named Peppy. He used to put me on him. Little did I know that one day cutting would become my passion.

Until I was sixteen years old, life seemed pretty ordinary. I showed in some local horse shows and did the typical teenage thing. My mother and I didn't get along for a while, and I even lost interest in the horses for a few years when I was in high school.

But then one day, when I was sixteen years old, a monster crept into our house and stole our security. For some reason, one morning my mother just couldn't get up off the couch anymore. She spent a year going through tests and was finally diagnosed with depression. It seemed to me like one day she was fine and the next day she was too ill to do anything. She had always been so active. Normally she would do ground-work with the colts Dad was training. She had a beautiful rose garden and was a mother and great horsewoman. Then one day—it was all gone. It made me sick.

The whole thing shook me up and made me worry that someday it could happen to me, although I swore it never would. I was proactive to keep myself mentally healthy and busy.

After high school I went off to college and tried to figure out who I was, and I guess I did. A few years later I returned to Washington State with a desire to get back to my roots. The first thing I did was buy a horse. I found a registered Quarter Horse named Pine Sprint, or Skippy. He was amazing. I could go out and herd cattle on him one day and the next day earn Western Pleasure points on him. He was happy, and I never had to worry about him. He was the kind of horse you only come across once in your lifetime. I bought him for my thirtieth birthday as a present to myself.

When Mom finally did get well from her depression, we drove around the county looking for a new horse for her. We all knew it was her best therapy. We found her a great little horse in Athol, Idaho, and she and I spent hours and hours in the saddle together—it was a wonderful bonding time for us. We hadn't gotten along when I was growing up, but after the depression, we became very close by riding horses together.

Skippy and I had several good years together, then I decided to become involved in cutting. It was time to move up to a new level of riding, so I bought a well-bred cutting horse I fondly called Little Buddy (Genuine Squaw Leo). He was in my price range, and I'd loved him ever since I met him at Golden West Quarter Horses in Washington. I started learning the basics of cutting on him. He was so handy and so nice—and he was a really pretty horse. I loved the sport, and I was having the time of my life.

But then, out of nowhere, I started having panic attacks.

My mom recognized my symptoms. By the time I went to a doctor, they realized that my thyroid was non-functional and I was anemic. Then I was diagnosed with depression. I was devastated. After all I had done to prevent the illness, there it was. Even though I knew the illness was genetic, I spent months feeling guilty about my condition and months finding the appropriate medications to set me right.

At this important juncture in my life, I realized how very much horses meant to me. Skippy and Buddy became my reason to get up each day. At first, it was hard to get myself going, but I knew I had to. I knew that my horses counted on me and that they had the ability to heal my damaged emotions. To keep myself going, I *had* to take care of the horses. By the time my medication got squared away, I *wanted* to go to the horses. Every ounce of my energy was focused on them. They were the best-groomed horses in the county, and their stalls were always picked perfectly clean.

A few years after I bought Buddy, my friends kept telling me it was time to move on—time to buy a more advanced horse if I were going to become a better cutter. So I bought Jewels Master Jay, a grandson of Colonel Freckles and Lenas Jewel Bars from Golden West Quarter Horses. "Little Jerry" was coming on three years old at the time, and he went straight into training. I loved his athletic ability. He was just a baby, but he had it all. After taking him to the Western Nationals in Ogden, Utah, just for the experience, I knew I had chosen the right horse. The warm-up arena was six horses deep, and he quickly learned how to be calm. Jerry and I were on our way.

But depression still continued to challenge me. My relationship soon started to fall apart because my partner didn't believe in depression. He thought I was just looking for attention. By this time, I had sold Buddy to my farrier, but I still owned Skippy. Between Little Jerry, Skippy, and my two border collies, I had plenty of therapy. My horses were my godsend. I love the smell of them and the hard work it takes to provide for them. Hard work is good for people with depression.

In 2007, when Skippy was twenty-eight years old, I had to put him down one evening. It was probably the worse day of my life. I was holding him in my lap when he died. I was in shock afterwards and slept on the couch in my jeans all that night. I couldn't take the jeans off because I could still smell him, and I never wanted to let go of that wonderful smell. He had gone down in the paddock and couldn't get up. I had called the vet out. It was not the way I wanted to say good-bye.

Losing Skippy was a powerful reminder to me of what all my horses have meant throughout the years. As I clung to my memories of him, I also clung to a profound sense of gratitude for a horse who had helped me live—who had been my life and my breath and my reason to keep going.

Five months later I had to put down the border collie who had been my companion for fourteen years. I immediately ran to my greatest source of comfort—Little Jerry. I knew he would understand.

As I look back at my overall "ride," I feel good. I went from riding a little black and white pony to competing at the Washington Cutting Horse Association. Depression was like a thief that crept into my life and stole my power. With the help of my horses, I took it back. Without even realizing they were doing it, they saved my life. And nobody will ever be able to take that away from me.